Aerobics Today

Aerobics Today

Carole Casten, Ph.D.
*California State University
Dominguez Hills*

Peg Jordan, R. N.
Aerobics and Fitness Association of America

Series Editor for West's Physical Activities Series

Robert J. O'Connor, Ed. D.
Los Angeles Pierce College

West Publishing Company
St. Paul   New York   Los Angeles   San Francisco

Cover Photo:	David Hanover Photography, Los Angeles, California
Intext Photos:	David Hanover Photography, Los Angeles, California
Additional Photos:	IDEA—The Association for Fitness Professionals
	Reebok, Inc.
	Aerobic Dancing, Inc.
	Body Focus
Composition:	Patti Zeman, Moorpark, California
Computer Illustration/ Production:	Miyake Illustration & Design, Moorpark, California

97 96 95 94 93 92 91 90   8 7 6 5 4 3 2 1 0

Library of Congress Cataloging-in-Publication Data

Casten, Carole M. Sokolow.
    Aerobics Today / Carole Casten, Peg Jordan.
    p. cm.—(West's Physical Activities Series)
    Includes bibliographical references.
    ISBN 0-314-68953-2
    1. Aerobic exercises.   I. Jordan, Peg.   II. Title.   III. Series.
RA781.15.C37   1990
613,7 ' 15—dc20   89–49155
                                                              CIP

Table of Contents

Preface   **ix**

Chapter 1   **Introduction**   **1**

Who Created Aerobics?   2
What Is Aerobics?   2
What Can We Expect to Gain from Aerobics?   3
Summary   3

Chapter 2   **Benefits of Aerobic Exercise**   **5**

Components of Fitness   6
Your Heart   8
Checklist for Taking Your Pulse   9
Frequency of Exercise   11
Intensity of Exercise   12
Duration of Exercise   12
Lifestyles and the Development of Cardiovacular Disease   12
Risko Factor Profile   13
Summary   17

Chapter 3   **Committing Yourself to a Workout**   **19**

Benefits of an Aerobic Dance Exercise Class   20
Components of a Good Class   20
Checklist for Your First Aerobic Class   21
Checklist for Warm-up   23
Frequency of Workouts   24
How Long Before Results Are Apparent?   24
What to Wear to Class   24
Selecting Shoes   24
Summary   26

Chapter 4   **Your Personal Workout**   **27**

Your Pre-Class Warm-up   28
Stretches and Isolations   28
Strengthening Exercises   37
Checklist for Your Personal Workout   43
Summary   44

Chapter 5   Motivation   45

Negative Motivation   46
Positive Motivation   47
Inner Directed versus Outer Directed   47
Why You Keep Going   48
Mental Benefits of Aerobics   48
Setting Goals   49
Following the Goals with Action   49
Visualization   49
Checklist for Mental Imaging   50
Additional Motivational Tips   50
Summary   50

Chapter 6   Body Composition and Weight Control   53

Basic Nutrition Guidelines   54
Checklist for Calories Contained in Four Food Groups   55
Weight Control   56
Body Composition   57
Checklist for Calculating Desirable Body Weight   58
Summary   58

Chapter 7   Injury Prevention   61

Prevention of Injury   62
Pain versus Exercise Discomfort   62
Treatment for Routine Injuries   62
Checklist for Treating Injuries   63
Overuse Injuries   63
Common Overuse Injuries   63
Common Causes of Aerobic Injuries   64
Summary   74

Chapter 8   Low-Impact Aerobics   75

Definition   76
Impact and Injuries   76
Protecting the Knees   77
Checklist for Knee Protection   77
Low-Back Precautions   77
The Questions of Weights   78
Low Impact versus Low Intensity   79
Aqua Exercise   79
Benefits   79
Summary   80

Chapter 9   Pregnancy and Dance Exercise   81

Value   82
Special Precautions   82
Modifications of an Aerobic Exercise Program   82

Special Exercises   86
Controversial Exercises   87
Exercises to Avoid   87
Summary   88

Chapter 10   Measuring Your Progress   89

What Condition Are You in Now   90
Assessing Your Personal Measurements   90
Testing Your Aerobic Capacity   92
Testing Your General Flexibility   94
Student Health History   95
Checklist: Semester Progress Chart   96
Summary   96

Chapter 11   Selecting a Class   97

What to Look for in a Good Instructor   98
Characteristics of a Good Instructor   98
The Aerobic Dance Exercise Class   98
Selecting a Facility   99
Checklist for Selecting a Facility   100
Summary   100

Chapter 12   A Guide to Buying Media for Personal Use   101

Selecting a Videotape to Use   102
Evaluating a Videotape   102
Checklist: Videotape Evaluation   102
Purchasing a Videotape   104
Selecting Music to Create Your Own Routines   104
Summary   104

Chapter 13   Being Creative: Choreographing Your Own Routines   105

Creating Your Own Dance Exercise Routines   106
Checklist: Creating a Routine   108
Simple 8-Count Movement Phrases   109
Summary   117

Chapter 14   Becoming An Instructor   119

Where to Study to Become an Instructor   120
Checklist: Do I Want to Be an Instructor?   121
Summary   121

Appendix A   Apparel   122

Appendix B   Associations and Organizations   125

Appendix C   Equipment   127

TABLE OF CONTENTS

Appendix D	**Books**	**130**
Appendix E	**Footwear**	**133**
Appendix F	**Music Videos**	**135**
Appendix G	**Sit and Reach Box**	**139**
Appendix H	**Miscellaneous**	**141**
Glossary		**143**
Index		**149**

Preface

AEROBICS TODAY is designed to assist the student of aerobic dance exercise. The text illustrates the benefits of aerobic dance exercise for levels of involvement from beginner to instructor with focus on understanding the basics. Careful attention has been given to laying the foundation for a safe and successful aerobic routine. Additionally, the authors have provided pertinent information with regard to pregnancy and exercise, the mental aspect of the sport, and information for would-be instructors.

The photographs clearly demonstrate how to properly perform exercises described in the book. These exercises have been found to be physically sound by exercise physiologists and recognized by certifying agencies.

The authors hope that AEROBICS TODAY will be a useful tool as you make aerobic dance a valuable part of your life.

To a healthy life!

Acknowledgements

The development of this text could not have progressed without the good advice and timely responses of the reviewers. The authors wish to thank the following colleagues for their input into the textbook:

Daniel Berney, *California State University, Dominguez Hills*
Sherri Hensley, *University of South Carolina*
Patrick Hodges, *Sinclair Community College*
Roberta Hopewell, *University of California at Riverside*
Tish Husak, *California State University, Long Beach*
Janice Lettunich, *University of Oregon*
Lisa Mazzeri, *Arizona State University*
Joan McPherson, *Southeast Missouri State University*
Debbie Powers, *Ball State University*

Dedication

I would like to dedicate this book to my daughter Kimberly, my husband Rich, and my mother. Without their support and patience, this book would not have been possible. I want to thank my co-author, Peg, for her friendship good humor, and good writing. My thanks also goes to Bob O'Connor for introducing me to West Publishing, and John Johnson for his confidence in my writing. Special thanks to the models used throughout the textbook: Maria Nilsson, Tim Plough, Renee Forrette, Florinda Tamada, Thyme Lewis, Laurie Botwinick, and Tom Smith. Thanks is also extended to the staff at West Educational Publishing, particularly to Mario Rodriguez and Theresa O'Dell, for their hard work on helping this project become a book.

Carole Casten, Ph.D.

The information I've shared in this book has been gathered from the innovative thinking and creations of Dr. Kenneth Cooper, Jacki Sorensen, and Marti Steele West. I dedicate this book to them, and their boundless aerobic energy. I would like to acknowledge Nancy Gillette and Linda Shelton for their contributions to injury prevention and safe instruction, and to Bonnie Rote for her work in prenatal exercise. My thanks go to my co-author Carole Casten, for her skilled teaching expertise and her lighthearted, positive attitude that overcame any obstacle to completing this project with me. I also want to thank Linda Pfeffer, President of the Aerobics and Fitness Association of America, for the opportunity to write for the organization.

Peg Jordan, RN

The Series Editor for West's Physical Activities Series

The Series Editor for West's Physical Activities Series is Dr. Bob O'Connor, Los Angeles Pierce College. Dr. O'Connor received his B.S. and M.S. degrees in physical education from UCLA and his doctorate from U.S.C. His 30-year teaching experience includes instruction in physical education courses of tennis, weight training, volleyball, badminton, swimming and various team sports, as well as classes in teaching methods. He brings to the Series a wide range of college coaching experience in areas of swimming, tennis, water polo, and football. Internationally, Dr. O'Connor has been an advisor to several Olympic programs in weight training and swimming. He was among the first to popularize strength training for all athletic events. Dr. O'Connor has written extensively in the fields of physical education and health and is a dedicated advocate of physical education TODAY.

Books in West's Physical Activities Series

Aerobics Today by Carole Casten and Peg Jordan
Badminton Today by Tariq Wadood and Karlyne Tan
Dance Today by Lorraine Person and Marian Weiser
Golf Today by J. C. Snead and John Johnson
Racquetball Today by Lynn Adams and Irwin Goldbloom
Swimming and Aquatics Today by Ron Ballatore and William Miller
Tennis Today by Glenn Bassett and William Otta
Volleyball Today by Marv Dunphy and Rod Wilde
Weight Training Today by Robert O'Connor, Jerry Simmons, and
J. Patrick O'Shea

CHAPTER 1

Introduction

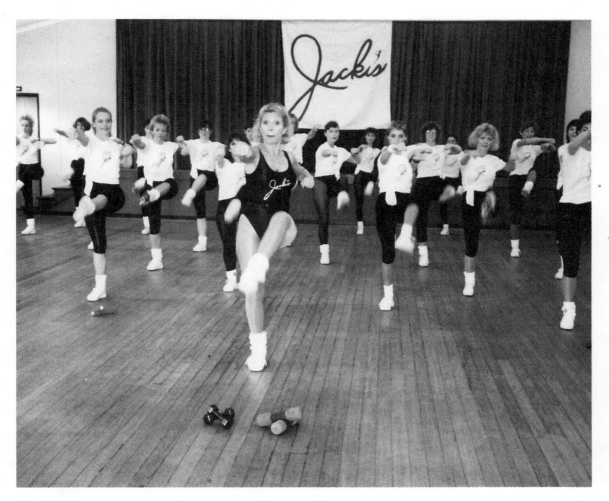

Outline

Who Created Aerobics?
What Is Aerobics?
What Can You Expect to Gain from Aerobics?
Summary

Aerobics, or dance exercise, is a popular form of exercise that incorporates a variety of dance movements performed to motivating music. Its purpose is to provide an enjoyable form of fitness development or exercise. More than 20 million people participate in aerobics annually. In fact, it is ranked as the sixth most popular activity in the nation according to H. R. Ritchie.

Who Created Aerobics?

Aerobic dance was created by Jacki Sorensen in 1969, a former dancer who believed in dance exercise as a beneficial form of achieving fitness. Dancercise, Jazzercise™, aerobics, and dance exercise are variations of her original work. Although each variation is slightly different, the basic formula for an aerobics class is the same: warm-up, cardiovascular work (aerobic exercise), specific muscular strength flexibility, and endurance work, and cool down.

What Is Aerobics?

The scientific definition for aerobic exercise is *exercise that utilizes oxygen for a sustained activity of two minutes or longer.* Today, aerobic dance exercise refers to dance movements that combine in a way to force the body to utilize oxygen for a sustained period of time.

Many people who find it boring to jog, bicycle, swim, or jump rope enjoy moving rhythmically to music. It is important to select a fitness activity or combination of activities that you enjoy so that you will stick with it. Gaining and maintaining fitness is a lifetime commitment.

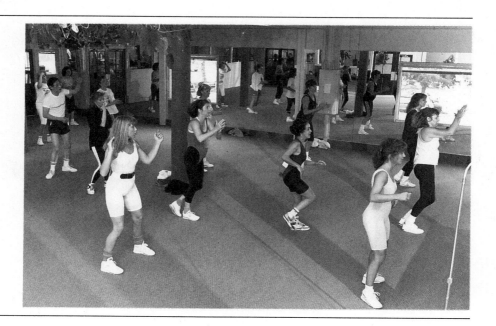

What Can You Expect to Gain from Aerobics?

People take aerobic dance exercise classes for many reasons. Some people like to dance and feel this is a good way to move to music, perform some dance steps, exercise, and have fun all at the same time. Others take aerobic dance exercise because they don't like to exercise outdoors, and this form of exercise usually is performed indoors. Still others participate in aerobics because their friends are doing it or to meet new people with similar interests.

Whatever your reason for doing aerobics, you can expect the following results if you attend a class three to five times a week for at least eight weeks. Though scientific research does not support all the following claims, people who regularly participate in aerobic dance exercise report that by following a regular exercise regime you will:

1. Have more energy.
2. Feel better about yourself.
3. Change your body composition by losing fat and increasing your lean body mass.
4. Look more toned.
5. Meet new people and make new friends.
6. Improve your digestion.
7. Improve the quality of your sleep.
8. Reduce your stress and the byproducts of stress.
9. Reduce your resting heart rate.
10. Improve your lung capacity.
11. Reduce the risk of cardiovascular disease.
12. Invoke a sense of discipline into your daily regimen.

Summary

1. Aerobic dance exercise was developed by Jacki Sorensen in 1969.
2. The format of aerobic classes has changed over the years as has its popularity. Today, more than 20 million people participate regularly in aerobic dance exercise.
3. Aerobic dance exercise is defined as dance movements combined in such a way as to cause the body to utilize oxygen for a sustained period of time.
4. To see results, it is important to participate in aerobic dance exercise for at least eight weeks, three to five times per week, at least fifty minutes per session.
5. The reasons people do aerobics instead of other forms of exercise vary greatly, from simply enjoying aerobics to being able to exercise with friends.
6. The benefits of participating in aerobic dance exercise include feeling better, looking better, losing weight, gaining muscle tone, reducing the resting heart rate, increasing lung capacity, gaining energy, and improving overall body fitness.

CHAPTER 2

Benefits of Aerobic Exercise

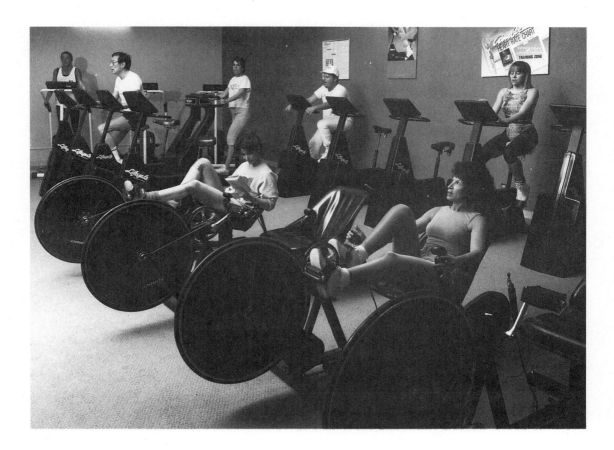

Outline

Components of Fitness
   Cardiovascular Efficiency
   Muscular Strength
   Muscular Endurance
   Flexibility
   Body Composition
Your Heart
   Resting Heart Rate
   Taking the Pulse
Checklist for Taking Your Pulse
   Target Heart Rate

The Karvonen Method
The American College of Sports
   Medicine Method
   Recovery Heart Rate
   Monitoring Your Heart Rate
Fluency of Exercise
Intensity of Exercise
Duration of Exercise
Lifestyles and the Development of
   Cardiovascular Disease
Risk Factor Profile
Risko Reference Charts
Summary

The benefits of aerobic exercise are numerous. Research has firmly established that regular, vigorous exercise is beneficial to the human body. One major benefit is that after exercising aerobically an individual feels "good" and exhilarated. Another benefit of aerobic exercise is a reduction of stress and tension in the body.

Also, coronary risk is lowered by increasing the beneficial type of cholesterol, high density lipoproteins (HDL) and reducing the ratio of total cholesterol to HDL. About 75 percent of your body's cholesterol is manufactured by the liver. The liver changes the cholesterol into low-density lipoproteins (LDLs) and triglylcerides. The LDLs and triglycerides enter the bloodstream and are deposited into various tissues. Excess LDL-cholesterol is deposited along arterial walls. This forms the plaque that blocks the bloodstream. Any HDLs in the area removes excess cholesterol from the bloodstream.

Other benefits of aerobic exercising are that muscle fibers get larger and perform more efficiently. Also, bones are strengthened, become more dense, and are more resistant to deterioration. Weight control is easier because aerobic exercise raises your metabolic rate, burning additional calories, increasing fat utilization and improving digestion and elimination. Additionally, the body becomes more physically fit. The heart muscle becomes stronger and more efficient and lung capacity increases. Muscles increase in strength and endurance and the body becomes more flexible. In short, aerobic exercise offers both psychological and physiological benefits.

Components of Fitness

An individual is considered to be physically fit when these five components of fitness are developed and balanced.

1. Cardiovascular fitness and efficiency
2. Muscular strength
3. Muscular endurance
4. Flexibility
5. Body composition

It is important that you understand these five components so that you know what is necessary to keep your body in top shape inside and outside.

Cardiovascular Efficiency

Cardiovascular efficiency and endurance refers to the body's ability to deliver oxygen to all of its vital organs. The efficiency of the heart and respiratory system determines how well the body provides oxygen to its vital organs during exercise and while at rest. The cardiovascular system consists of the heart, lungs, and blood vessels. At all times, but particularly during the stress of exercise, the cardiovascular system must be able to transport oxygen efficiently to provide the needed energy to the heart, lungs and working muscles. An efficient cardiovascular system is essential to a high level of physical fitness. Exercise increases the strength of the heart, which increases its ability to pump blood most efficiently throughout the body.

Cardiovascular endurance, or aerobic fitness, is the ability of the heart and respiratory system to deliver blood and therefore oxygen to the working muscles during prolonged exercise.

Muscular Strength

Muscular strength is the amount of force produced when a muscle group contracts and moves a resistance one time. Strength is essential to a variety of everyday activities such as lifting and moving objects; opening doors, jars, and windows; carrying children; and walking up stairs. Muscular strength is increased when the muscle is overloaded by repetitive activities and/or when a resistance or weight is added to the muscle. (A resistance is any amount of additional weight the body moves.)

Muscular Endurance

Muscular endurance is the ability of the muscles to exert force over an extended period of time. Endurance is an important element in helping you participate in repetitive activities, such as aerobics, jogging, swimming, walking, dancing, and stair climbing.

Flexibility

Flexibility is the range of motion possible in the joints. Flexibility is necessary to maintain body mobility. The more flexible you are, the more easily you can move your limbs through their full range of motion. The more flexible your muscles are, the fewer sore muscles and joint injuries you will have. Inactivity can produce the effect of tightening or shortening the muscles, thereby yielding a greater risk of injury when the muscles are put to use or stressed even a little.

Body Composition

Body composition is the relation of body fat to lean body mass (muscle, bone, cartilage, vital organs). To be considered lean, women must have less than 22 percent of their weight in fat and men must have less than 15 percent.

We are all born with a genetically determined body type. There are three kinds of **body types** or **somatotypes**: mesomorph, endomorph, and ectomorph. The mesomorph is characterized as having a predominance of muscle and bone and is often labeled "very muscular looking." Mesomorphic body types perform best in activities requiring strength, speed, and agility. The endomorph is a soft and round-looking individual with an excess of adipose or fatty tissue. Endomorphic body types have difficulty performing aerobic and skill-oriented activities. Ectomorphic body types are very thin and lean. These people do well in endurance activities such as aerobics but may have difficulty in activities requiring strength.

Don't fret if you don't fit into one body-type classification. Very few people are classified as being one somatotype. Usually a person is a combination of types (such as the mesomorphic endomorph, who appears muscular yet has a rounded look). The importance of knowing this information is that we are all different. Your goal must be personal. Your objective should be to be the best you can, with the body you inherited.

It is important to the quality of your life and health that you be at least minimally fit in each of the components of fitness. A person who is minimally physically fit has enough strength and endurance to perform daily tasks without undue fatigue and has enough energy left to enjoy leisure activity and be able to deal with an emergency situation.

Somatotypes

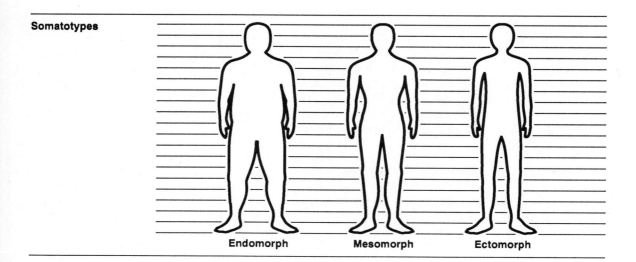

| Endomorph | Mesomorph | Ectomorph |

Your Heart

Scientific evidence indicates that regular cardiovascular exercise strengthens the heart muscle and reduces the risk of cardiovascular problems. Through exercise overload, the heart muscle becomes more fit and is able to work more efficiently and effectively. Exercise overload occurs when the body is subjected to greater exercise stress than it is accustomed to. When you perform exercise overload in a progressive and moderate amount, you strengthen muscles. However, if exercise overload is done in a nonprogressive, uncontrolled, and excessive manner, injury might occur. The more fit the heart is, the more oxygen-carrying blood can be pumped to the body with each contraction of the heart. Thus, a fit heart does not need to work as hard or beat as frequently as a less fit heart. In discussing cardiovascular fitness and efficiency, you need to be aware of your resting heart rate, your target heart rate, and your recovery heart rate.

Resting Heart Rate

Resting heart rate refers to the number of times your heart beats per minute upon waking or when you have been sitting or resting for approximately ten minutes. The best time to take your resting heart rate is when you first wake up and are still lying down. To obtain the most accurate reading, take your pulse for sixty seconds on two consecutive mornings, and then average the two numbers. A person who exercises regularly may have a lower resting heart rate than a person who is sedentary. An average resting heart rate is about 72 beats per minute. If you discover your resting heart rate has decreased after you've done a few months of regular aerobic exercise, it indicates you are getting fit. That's a sign you would like to see.

Taking the Pulse

For most people, taking the pulse is easiest at the carotid artery. The carotid pulse is located in the groove of the neck, next to the Adam's apple. Use your first two fingers and press lightly on the carotid artery (be careful not to press too hard). You will feel your pulse.

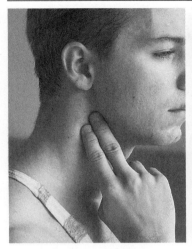
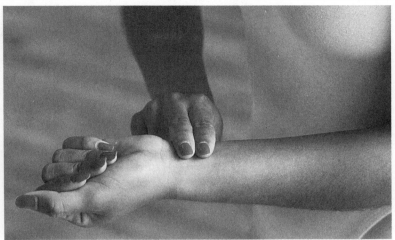

Pulse at the carotid artery   **Pulse at the radial artery**

Another place to take your pulse is at the radial artery (on the thumb side of your wrist, palm up). When taking your pulse, be sure to use the first two or three fingers, not the thumb. The thumb has a pulse of its own and therefore could cause an inaccurate reading.

Checklist for Taking Your Pulse

1. With your index and middle fingers (not your thumb) you can find your pulse in the carotid artery very easily:

   Place you fingers on your Adam's apple. Gently slide your fingers toward the outside of the neck, into the natural "notch" on the side of your neck. By pressing lightly, you can feel the pulse at the carotid artery.

2. You can find your radial pulse by:

   Placing your fingers lightly on the inside of your wrist. To do this, rotate one arm in so the palm of your hand is facing you. Then place the fingers of the opposite hand just above your wrist on the thumb side of your arm and just inside the arm bone (the radius). You will feel the radial pulse.

3. Count the number of pulse beats for a minute. You can do this by:
   - Counting your pulse for 30 seconds and multiplying by 2.
   - Counting your pulse for 15 seconds and multiplying by 4.
   - Counting your pulse for 10 seconds and multiplying by 6.

   The 10 second count is preferred when you are taking your pulse during exercise.

Target Heart Rate

Target heart rate (THR) is the level at which you will gain the benefits of exercising your heart to improve cardiovascular fitness. There are two accepted formulas for calculating your target heart rate. Use both formulas. Compare the two results, and choose the level where you will work. (You may choose an average of the two results.)

You need to first determine the intensity level at which you would like to work. A person who has been sedentary for a long time may want to begin an exercise regimen at the 60 percent level and work up gradually to 70 percent. It is generally accepted that for most people, 70 percent is a good level at which to work. Athletes and highly fit individuals may work at 85 percent.

Second, you must determine your resting heart rate. Once you determine your intensity level and your resting heart rate, proceed with the following formulas.

The Karvonen Method

The **Karvonen method** of determining the target heart rate for a 20-year-old person working at 70 percent intensity is as follows:

THR = Target Heart Rate
MHR = Maximum Heart Rate
RHR = Resting Heart Rate

THR = (MHR – RHR) x .70 + RHR

220 *minus* age = maximum heart rate (MHR)	220 – 20 = 200
200 *minus* resting heart rate (RHR) = heart rate range	200 – 80 = 120
120 *times* the desired intensity of activity (70%)	120 x .70 = 84
Heart rate range *plus* the resting heart rate beats per minute	84 + 80 = 164

164 = target heart rate (THR)

Divide the target heart rate by 6 to get the number you need for a 10-second pulse count: 164 ÷ 6 = 27

The American College of Sports Medicine Method

The American College of Sports Medicine recommends a simpler formula. Just subtract your age from 220, multiply by the desired intensity of your workout level, and divide the answer by 6 for a 10-second pulse estimate. It is recommended that your working target heart rate be 65 to 85 percent of your maximum heart rate.

The following example is again for a 20-year old working at the 70 percent level.

220 *minus* 20	= 200	Maximum heart rate
200 *times* .7	= 140	Target heart rate (THR)
140 *divided* by 6 =	23	Number of pulse beats in a 10-second period

To work at the desired level of intensity, this 20-year old would consider the results of both formulas and strive for 23 to 27 pulse beats during a 10-second count.

Be careful not to work over your target heart rate for more than a few seconds. You will not get into shape any faster. Working over your target heart rate may fatigue you faster, cause you discomfort, and even be unhealthy for you. Use common sense to check your exertion: if you are feeling extreme fatigue, you are probably overworking yourself.

Recovery Heart Rate

Your recovery heart rate is how quickly your pulse returns to normal after an aerobic workout. The more aerobically conditioned you are, the faster your heart will return to normal, or recover. Take your pulse two to five minutes after exercising. Your heart rate should be below 100 beats per minute.

Recovery Heart Rate Chart

Take your pulse 2 to 5 minutes after exercising. If you have a decrease from your target heart rate of

60 beats per minute = Super Recovery Rate
50 beats per minute = Excellent Recovery Rate
40 beats per minute = Good
30 beats per minute = Acceptable

After several months of consistently working out aerobically, you may notice that your heart rate recovers faster and is lower than before you began your exercise regimen. Your heart rate should return to its pre-exercise level within ten minutes after class ends. If it doesn't, you may have over-exerted yourself during the aerobics portion of class. Reduce the intensity of your workout during the next class, and monitor the length of time it takes for your heart rate to return to normal.

Monitoring Your Heart Rate

Monitoring your heart rate during exercise is extremely important. Take your pulse several times during, and especially immediately following, the aerobics portion of class. Your instructor will most likely lead the group, but if not, monitor your heart rate yourself. You need to make sure you are working within your appropriate target heart rate zone. If, when checking your pulse, you discover you are working at too high a level, adjust your movements to reduce the intensity of the workout. To reduce the intensity of exercise, keep your arms lower than your heart and don't lift your legs as high as you did previously. If you find you are not working as high as your target heart rate, increase your workload by making larger movements or lifting your arms or legs higher. However, never lift your legs higher than hip level.

Frequency of Exercise .

Frequency of exercise refers to how often you exercise per week. To obtain benefits from working out, you should participate in the aerobic portion of class three to five times a week for twenty to thirty minutes per session. If you exercise only once a week, you do not improve your fitness level, and you will probably be sore after exercising because of the stress you have placed on unconditioned muscles. Exercising every day is not necessary either. Studies show that people who rest at least one day a week have fewer injuries than those who exercise daily. Similarly, exercising three to five times a week appears to be as beneficial as exercising six or seven days a week. The body needs time to rest and recuperate so that you can avoid strained muscles and shin splints. An occasional day off is of great value in developing and maintaining fitness, both physically and psychologically.

Intensity of Exercise

Intensity of exercise refers to how hard you work when exercising. Once you have identified your target heart rate, you should continually monitor the intensity at which you are working. Working too hard is ineffective, as it can make you sore and may result in an injury. The key is to find the optimal level of intensity for your body and to meet your goals.

Duration of Exercise

Duration of exercise refers to how long you work out at one time. The duration of your exercise sessions depends on the components of fitness you are trying to develop.

You must spend time on each component of fitness you are trying to develop as well as time on each muscle group. For each component, you must do at least five continuous minutes of exercise at one time. For the cardiovascular component, you must do a minimum of twenty continuous minutes of concentrated effort in your target heart rate zone. As mentioned earlier, a fifty-minute aerobic dance exercise class that meets three to five times per week provides you with a good duration of exercise weekly to meet most of your goals.

Lifestyles and the Development of Cardiovascular Disease

Studies show that certain attributes, habits, and styles of living have a high degree of correlation with the development of cardiovascular disease. Factors known to increase the risks of cardiovascular disease are: a family history of heart disease; high blood pressure; cigarette smoking; being overweight; high levels of triglycerides and cholesterol in the blood; diabetes; stress; and physical inactivity.

An analysis of your personal risk factors will guide you toward achieving a healthy lifestyle. To perform a self-analysis, complete the following Risk Factor Profile.

RISKO Factor Profile

Instructions: To determine your score, circle the appropriate numbers to the right of each item that applies to you. Then add your score up and check your risk analysis against the scoring list.

MEN: Find the column for your age group. Everyone starts with a score of 10 points. Work down the page adding points to your score or subtracting points from your score.

		54 or Younger		54 or Older	
1. WEIGHT		**Starting Score**	**10**	**Starting Score**	**10**
Locate your weight category in the table below. If you are in . . .	weight category A	Subtract 2		Subtract 2	
	weight category B	Subtract 1		Subtract 0	
	weight category C	Add 1		Add 1	
	weight category D	Add 2		Add 3	
2. SYSTOLIC BLOOD PRESSURE		**Equals**		**Equals**	
Use the "first" or "higher" number from your most recent blood pressure measurement. If you do not know your blood pressure, estimate it by using the letter for your weight category. If your blood pressure is . . .	A 119 or less	Subtract 1		Subtract 5	
	B between 120 and 139	Add 0		Subtract 2	
	C between 140 and 159	Add 0		Add 1	
	D 160 or greater	Add 1		Add 4	
3. BLOOD CHOLESTEROL LEVEL		**Equals**		**Equals**	
Use the number from your most recent blood cholesterol test. If you do not know your blood cholesterol, estimate it by using the letter for your weight category. If your blood cholesterol is . . .	A 199 or less	Subtract 2		Subtract 1	
	B between 200 and 224	Subtract 1		Subtract 1	
	C between 225 and 249	Add 0		Add 0	
	D 250 or higher	Add 1		Add 0	
4. CIGARETTE SMOKING		**Equals**		**Equals**	
If you . . . *(If you smoke a pipe, but not cigarettes, use the same score adjustment as those cigarette smokers who smoke less than a pack a day.)*	do not smoke	Subtract 1		Subtract 2	
	smoke less than a pack a day	Add 0		Subtract 1	
	smoke a pack a day	Add 1		Add 0	
	smoke more than a pack a day	Add 2		Add 3	
		Final Score Equals		**Final Score Equals**	

WEIGHT TABLE FOR MEN	Your Height		Weight Category (lbs.)			
	Ft.	In.	A	B	C	D
Look for your height (without shoes) in the far left column and then read across to find the category into which your weight (in indoor clothing) would fall.	5	1	up to 123	124–148	149–173	174 plus
	5	2	up to 126	127–152	153–178	179 plus
	5	3	up to 129	130–156	157–182	183 plus
	5	4	up to 132	133–160	161–186	187 plus
	5	5	up to 135	136–163	164–190	191 plus
	5	6	up to 139	140–168	169–196	197 plus
	5	7	up to 144	145–174	175–203	204 plus
	5	8	up to 148	149–179	180–209	210 plus
	5	9	up to 152	153–184	185–214	215 plus
	5	10	up to 157	158–190	191–221	222 plus
	5	11	up to 161	162–194	195–227	228 plus
	6	0	up to 165	166–199	200–232	233 plus
	6	1	up to 170	171–205	206–239	240 plus
Because both blood pressure and blood cholesterol are related to weight, an estimate of these risk factors for each weight category is printed at the bottom of the table.	6	2	up to 175	176–211	212–246	247 plus
	6	3	up to 180	181–217	218–253	254 plus
	6	4	up to 185	186–223	224–260	261 plus
	6	5	up to 190	191–229	230–267	268 plus
	6	6	up to 195	196–235	236–274	275 plus
Estimate of Systolic Blood Pressure			119 or less	120 to 139	140 to 159	160 or more
Estimate of Blood Cholesterol			199 or less	200 to 224	225 to 249	250 or more

WOMEN: Find the column for your age group. Everyone starts with a score of 10 points. Work down the page adding points to your score or subtracting points from your score.

		54 or Younger	54 or Older

1. WEIGHT

Locate your weight category in the table below. If you are in . . .

	54 or Younger	54 or Older
	Starting Score 10	**Starting Score** 10
weight category A	Subtract 2	Subtract 2
weight category B	Subtract 1	Subtract 1
weight category C	Add 1	Add 1
weight category D	Add 2	Add 1

2. SYSTOLIC BLOOD PRESSURE   Equals ☐   Equals ☐

Use the "first" or "higher" number from your most recent blood pressure measurement. If you do not know your blood pressure, estimate it by using the letter for your weight category. If your blood pressure is . . .

		54 or Younger	54 or Older
A	119 or less	Subtract 2	Subtract 3
B	between 120 and 139	Subtract 1	Add 0
C	between 140 and 159	Add 0	Add 3
D	160 or greater	Add 2	Add 6

3. BLOOD CHOLESTEROL LEVEL   Equals ☐   Equals ☐

Use the number from your most recent blood cholesterol test. If you do not know your blood cholesterol, estimate it by using the letter for your weight category. If your blood cholesterol is . . .

		54 or Younger	54 or Older
A	199 or less	Subtract 1	Subtract 3
B	between 200 and 224	Add 0	Subtract 1
C	between 225 and 249	Add 0	Add 1
D	250 or higher	Add 1	Add 3

4. CIGARETTE SMOKING   Equals ☐   Equals ☐

If you . . .

	54 or Younger	54 or Older
do not smoke	Subtract 1	Subtract 2
smoke less than a pack a day	Add 0	Subtract 1
smoke a pack a day	Add 1	Add 1
smoke more than a pack a day	Add 2	Add 4
	Final Score Equals ☐	**Final Score Equals** ☐

WEIGHT TABLE FOR WOMEN

	Your Height		Weight Category (lbs.)			
	Ft.	In.	A	B	C	D
Look for your height (without shoes) in the far left column and then read across to find the category into which your weight (in indoor clothing) would fall.	4	8	up to 101	102–122	123–143	144 plus
	4	9	up to 103	104–125	126–146	147 plus
	4	10	up to 106	107–128	129–150	151 plus
	4	11	up to 109	110–132	133–154	155 plus
	5	0	up to 112	113–136	137–158	159 plus
	5	1	up to 115	116–139	140–162	163 plus
	5	2	up to 119	120–144	145–168	169 plus
	5	3	up to 122	123–148	149–172	173 plus
	5	4	up to 127	128–154	155–179	180 plus
	5	5	up to 131	132–158	159–185	186 plus
	5	6	up to 135	136–163	164–190	191 plus
	5	7	up to 139	140–168	169–196	197 plus
	5	8	up to 143	144–173	174–202	203 plus
Because both blood pressure and blood cholesterol are related to weight, an estimate of these risk factors for each weight category is printed at the bottom of the table.	5	9	up to 147	148–178	179–207	208 plus
	5	10	up to 151	152–182	183–213	214 plus
	5	11	up to 155	156–187	188–218	219 plus
	6	0	up to 159	160–191	192–224	225 plus
	6	1	up to 163	164–196	197–229	230 plus
Estimate of Systolic Blood Pressure			119 or less	120 to 139	140 to 159	160 or more
Estimate of Blood Cholesterol			199 or less	200 to 224	225 to 249	250 or more

WHAT YOUR SCORE MEANS

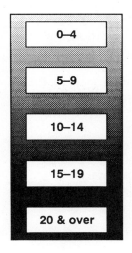

0–4
5–9
10–14
15–19
20 & over

You have one of the lowest risks of heart disease for your age and sex.

You have a low to moderate risk of heart disease for your age and sex but there is some room for improvement.

You have a moderate to high risk of heart disease for your age and sex, with considerable room for improvement on some factors.

You have a high risk of developing heart disease for your age and sex with a great deal of room for improvement on all factors.

You have a very high risk of developing heart disease for your age and sex and should take immediate action on all risk factors.

WARNING

- If you have diabetes, gout or a family history of heart disease, your actual risk will be greater than indicated by this appraisal.
- If you do not know your current blood pressure or blood cholesterol level, you should visit your physician or health center to have them measured. Then figure your score again for a more accurate determination of your risk.
- If you are overweight, have high blood pressure or high blood cholesterol, or smoke cigarettes: your long-term risk of heart disease is increased even if your risk in the next several years is low.

HOW TO REDUCE YOUR RISK

- Try to quit smoking permanently. There are many programs available.
- Have your blood pressure checked regularly, preferably every twelve months after age 40. If your blood pressure is high, see your physician. Remember blood pressure medicine is only effective if taken regularly.
- Consider your daily exercise (or lack of it). A half hour of brisk walking, swimming or other enjoyable activity should not be difficult to fit into your day.
- Give some serious thought to your diet. If you are overweight, or eat a lot of foods high in saturated fat or cholesterol (whole milk, cheese, eggs, butter, fatty foods, fried foods) then changes should be made in your diet. Look for the American Heart Association Cookbook at your local bookstore.
- Visit or write your local Heart Association for further information and copies of free pamphlets on many related subjects including:
  - Reducing your risk of heart attack.
  - Controlling high blood pressure.
  - Eating to keep your heart healthy.
  - How to stop smoking.
  - Exercising for good health.

SOME WORDS OF CAUTION

- If you have diabetes, gout, or a family history of heart disease, your real risk of developing heart disease will be greater than indicated by your RISKO score. If your score is high and you have one or more of these additional problems, you should give particular attention to reducing your risk.
- If you are a woman under 45 years or a man under 35 years of age, your RISKO score represents an upper limit on your real risk of developing heart disease. In this case, your real risk is probably lower than indicated by your score.
- Using your weight category to estimate your systolic blood pressure or your blood cholesterol level makes your RISKO score less accurate.
- Your score will tend to overestimate your risk if your actual values on these two important factors are average for someone of your height and weight.
- Your score will underestimate your risk if your actual blood pressure or cholesterol level is above average for someone of your height or weight.

UNDERSTANDING HEART DISEASE

In the United States it is estimated that close to 550,000 people die each year from coronary heart disease. Coronary artery disease is the most common type of heart disease and the leading cause of death in the United States and many other countries.

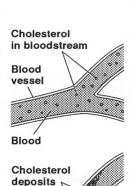

Cholesterol in bloodstream

Blood vessel

Blood

Cholesterol deposits

Coronary heart disease is the result of coronary atherosclerosis. Coronary atherosclerosis is the name of the process by which an accumulation of fatty deposits leads to a thickening and narrowing of the inner walls of the arteries that carry oxygenated blood and nutrients to the heart muscle. The effect is similar to that of a water pipe clogged by deposits.

The resulting restriction of the blood supply to the heart muscle can cause injury to the muscle as well as angina (chest pain). If the restriction of the blood supply is severe or if it continues over a period of time, the heart muscle cells fed by the restricted artery suffer irreversible injury and die. This is known as a myocardial infarction or heart attack.

Scientists have identified a number of factors which are linked with an increased likelihood or risk of developing coronary heart disease. Some of these risk factors, like aging, being male, or having a family history of heart disease, are unavoidable. However, many other significant risk factors, including all of the factors used to determine your RISKO score, can be changed to reduce the likelihood of developing heart disease.

APPRAISING YOUR RISK

- The RISKO heart hazard appraisal is an indicator of risk for adults who do not currently show evidence of heart disease. However, if you already have heart disease, it is very important that you work with your doctor in reducing your risk.
- The original concept of RISKO was developed by the Michigan Heart Association.
- It has been further developed by the American Heart Association with the assistance of Drs. John and Sonja McKinlay in Boston. It is based on the Framingham, Stanford, and Chicago heart disease studies. The format of RISKO was tested and refined by Dr. Robert M. Chamberlain and Dr. Armin Weinberg of the National Heart Center at the Baylor College of Medicine in

Summary

1. Research has established that regular, vigorous exercise is beneficial to the human body in many ways. The benefits are as follows:
   - An individual feels good after exercising aerobically.
   - Stress and tension in the body are reduced.
   - Coronary heart disease risk is lowered.
   - Muscle fibers perform more efficiently.
   - Bones are strengthened.
   - Weight control is easier because aerobic exercise raises your metabolic rate and allows you to burn more calories.
   - The heart muscle becomes stronger and more efficient.

2. Five components of fitness are:
   - Cardiovascular efficiency.
   - Muscular strength.
   - Muscular endurance.
   - Flexibility.
   - Body composition.

3. To understand your cardiovascular fitness and efficiency, you must be aware of and know how to calculate your:
   - Resting heart rate.
   - Target heart rate.
   - Maximum heart rate.
   - Recovery heart rate.

4. You can take your pulse easily by using the carotid or the radial pulse.

5. The minimum number of times you need to exercise in order to achieve aerobic benefits is three sessions per week.
   - For greater aerobic benefit, exercise five times per week.
   - Participating in a fifty-minute to sixty-minute aerobic dance class three to five times per week will help you meet most of your fitness goals.

6. To get the proper duration of exercise:
   - You must do at least five continuous minutes of exercise at one time for each component of fitness.
   - You must do a minimum of twenty continuous minutes of concentrated effort, in your target heart rate zone, for the cardiovascular component.

7. Factors known to increase the risks of cardiovascular disease are:
   - A family history of heart disease.
   - High blood pressure.
   - Cigarette smoking.
   - Being overweight.
   - High levels of triglycerides and cholesterol in the blood.
   - Diabetes.
   - Stress
   - Physical inactivity.

CHAPTER 3

Committing Yourself to a Workout

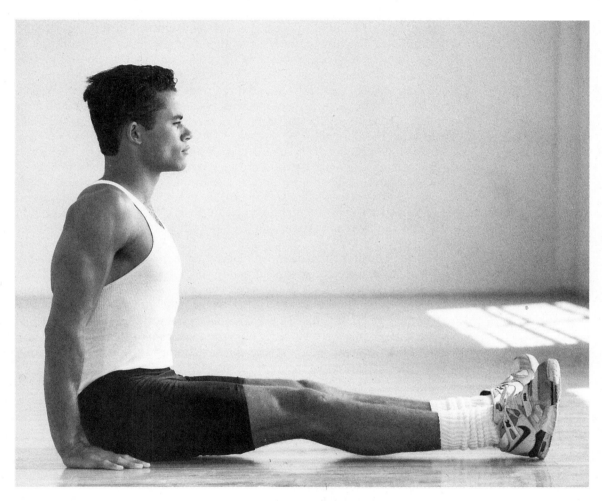

Outline

Benefits of an Aerobic Dance Exercise Class
Components of a Good Class
Checklist for Your First Aerobics Class
    Warm-Up and Stretching
    Cardiovascular/Aerobics Work
    Strengthening and Toning Work
    Cool-Down and Flexibility
Checklist for Warm-Up
Frequency of Workouts
How Long Before Results Are Apparent
What to Wear to Class
Selecting Shoes
Summary

To get the benefit from exercising and from aerobics specifically, you *must* stick with it! Exercising must become an integral part of your weekly routine. You need to be convinced of the benefits you will derive from it, and then you will make exercising a part of your lifestyle. Schedule your aerobics class into your life, and don't allow other things to interrupt this commitment.

Benefits of an Aerobic Dance Exercise Class

There are physiological, psychological, and social benefits of an aerobic dance exercise class. The physiological benefits, as discussed in the last chapter, are numerous. The heart muscle strengthens and becomes more efficient as it pumps more blood. Lung capacity increases, and muscle fibers increase in size and perform more efficiently. The number of red blood cells increases. Bones become stronger, denser, and more resistant to deterioration. Weight control is aided because the metabolic rate is elevated for several hours after exercise, and more calories are burned during exercise. Also, digestion and elimination are improved.

A psychological benefit is a feeling of well-being after exercise. Research suggests that during exercise a euphoria-producing chemical called enkephalin is released. Brain cells release similar substances called endorphins, which produce a feeling of well-being and relaxation. In addition, you feel better when you know you are doing something good for yourself. Once you start looking better and seeing results from exercise you will feel better during and after class.

A social benefit is that you meet people in an aerobic dance class. Having familiar faces and people to talk to before and after a class helps keep you motivated to continue exercising. Also, you receive emotional support from your friends to continue your exercise program. You know the saying, "misery loves company." If you miss an aerobics class, you can be sure someone will ask you where you were. Another important social aspect is that exercising is more fun in groups. If you are having fun exercising, you are more likely to make the activity a regular part of your life.

Components of a Good Class

All good aerobics or dance exercise classes have four parts:
1. Warm-up and stretching.
2. Cardiovascular/aerobics work.
3. Strengthening and toning work.
4. Cool-down and flexibility.

It is important to participate in all four parts of the class as they are designed to prepare your body for the work you are doing in a progressive, safe, manner. Also, to get the best results from working out, you need to work on all components of conditioning.

Many people associate a good workout with pain. You've heard the phrase "no pain, no gain." Such an erroneous concept is reinforced by popular media. You will experience some discomforts during and after a good class—some mild aches and soreness, perhaps a slight shortness of breath, and a feeling of fatigue. But these discomforts are minor and temporary. Be careful, because

Checklist for Your First Aerobics Class

1. Are you the type of person who sticks to something from the start, or do you drop out before the job is done? If you are the former, then you will easily commit yourself to a workout.
2. To benefit from exercise, you must stick with it.
3. Make a schedule of your weekly commitments. Find a window of time to fit regular exercise into your schedule.
4. The three facets of life where aerobic dance exercise will benefit you are in the physiological, psychological, and social parts of your life.
5. The four components of a good class are:
   • Warm-up and stretching
   • Aerobics/cardiovascular work
   • Strengthening and toning work
   • Cool down and flexibility
6. Remember, "No pain, no gain" is an erroneous concept.
7. You should workout 3 to 5 times per week at such an adequate intensity as to achieve cardiovascular fitness.
8. Do not become discouraged, remember that it will take approximately 8 weeks to see the visible results of your hard work through exercise.
9. Wear comfortable clothes to class that allow your body to breath. Do not wear nylon, rubber, or non-permeable clothes.
10. Select shoes that are meant for aerobic exercising. They should be comfortable, provide you with good support and have impact-absorption qualities.

if you feel pain when you exercise, this is a sign of over-exercising (or over-exertion), and you need to moderate your activity. A good aerobics class offers activities that will not hurt you. However, you must always protect yourself and understand and respect the signs your body gives you.

Warm-Up and Stretching

The warm-up portion of class usually lasts seven to ten minutes. The purpose is to activate your circulatory system and progressively prepare your body for the upcoming high-intensity activities. During warm-up, your heart rate gradually increases, circulation improves, ventilation increases, oxygen flow increases, muscles and joints warm up and become more flexible, stiffness and soreness are reduced. Additionally, a warm-up mentally prepares you to participate fully in the dance exercise class. Tension gradually subsides during that time because of the rhythmic movement.

The warm-up also includes stretching. It is very important that you perform static stretches (or stretches that are sustained for a period of time without extra movement) and that you hold your stretches. Do not participate in bouncing, or what is called ballistic stretching. Ballistic stretching can lead to the tearing of muscles. Each person has a different degree of flexibility. Know your capabilities and be aware of your limitations. If you feel discomfort or extreme tightness, release the stretch you are in and do not stretch any further in that position.

Another very important point to remember is that when you warm your body up progressively and properly, you reduce the potential for injury. It is imperative that you arrive on time to your aerobics class so that you don't miss the warm-up.

Cardiovascular/Aerobics Work

The aerobic portion of the class begins slowly and progressively increases in intensity to gradually overload your circulatory system. The length varies from 12 to 30 minutes depending on the overall length and level of the class. The aerobic routines incorporate a variety of movements designed to use all parts of the body and to raise the heart rate to its target zone. Between movement phases, or every 5 to 10 minutes, monitor your pulse to determine if you are working at the correct intensity to maintain your target heart rate.

The purpose of the cardiovascular/aerobic phase of class is to:

1. Elevate the heart rate to the target zone, and keep it there for 12 to 30 minutes.
2. Strengthen the heart muscle.
3. Stress the circulatory system, which yields cardiovascular endurance.
4. Improve and increase muscular endurance.
5. Improve and increase lung ventilation.

A post-aerobic cool-down is extremely important. It is wise to end the aerobic section of class with approximately 2 to 3 minutes of slower-paced movements. During this period, the heart rate and blood pressure return to a more stable level before you proceed to floor work. At the end of this brief cool-down period, your heart rate should be at or under 60 percent of your maximum heart rate.

Strengthening and Toning Work

A good instructor makes a smooth transition to the floor to begin strengthening and conditioning. The purpose of this phase, which lasts approximately 10 to 20 minutes, is to increase the strength, endurance, tone, and flexibility of your muscles. A good instructor leads exercises that work the entire body. A concentrated effort is made to increase the muscular strength and endurance of the biceps, triceps, thighs, abdomen, abdominal muscles, and buttocks (gluteals).

Upon approaching the floor, you may find yourself a little light-headed. If so, tell your instructor. You may need to walk around the room a while in order to lower your heart rate more gradually.

Cool-Down and Flexibility

The purpose of the cool-down and flexibility phase is to allow the body to gradually recover from the stress placed on it during your high-intensity workout. Cooling down has two parts:

1. To ease you out of your aerobic and strengthening activity at a slow pace in order to allow your heart rate to return to normal.
2. To stretch your muscles so that injury and stiffening are prevented. If you stop exercising suddenly, you may cause a pooling of blood in the lower legs. This may result in dizziness or a light-headed feeling.

At the end of class, you should perform slow, steady stretching for a minimum of 5 minutes to redistribute the blood flow equally and return the body to its pre-exercise state. After 5 to 10 minutes of cool-down, your heart rate should be close to 100 beats per minute. Remember that warm muscles stretch best. Perform static stretches and hold all of your stretches for approximately 10 to 30 seconds.

 ## Checklist for Warm-Up

Begin your warm-up activities with a progressively paced, gentle form of aerobic activity to "start your circulation moving," so to speak. For example, you could begin by slowly walking around the room and gradually walking faster until you reach a jogging pace. You could also increase your heart rate by performing jumping jacks or running in place slowly to music. Continue this type of overall body warm-up for approximately two to three minutes. Then begin stretching activities. A well-designed aerobics class incorporates this type of warm-up into the early part of the class.

Stretching
Stretch each large muscle group in your body slowly. Hold each stretch for approximately 20 seconds.

1. Legs
    ___ Hamstrings (back of the thighs)
    ___ Quadriceps (front of the thighs)
    ___ Abductors (outside of the thighs and hips)
    ___ Adductors (inside of the thighs and hips)
    ___ Gastrocnemius (calf muscle)
    ___ Tibialis anterior (muscle in front of leg, below the knee)

2. Back
    ___ Upper back
    ___ Lower back

3. Abdominals
    ___ Front
    ___ Sides

4. Shoulders

5. Neck

Frequency of Workouts

Research indicates that working out with adequate intensity three to five times per week is all that is necessary to achieve cardiovascular fitness. You don't have to knock yourself out seven days per week. It is important physiologically and psychologically to allow yourself a 24- to 48-hour recovery each week. Attending an aerobics class three to five times per week will keep you in good shape.

How Long Before Results Are Apparent?

Improved fitness and changes in your appearance take time. So don't become discouraged if you don't see a change in your body after only one week of working out. Research indicates that people participating in a vigorous physical exercise program experience increased efficiency in their cardiovascular system in approximately eight weeks. However, after a few weeks, you will notice an improvement in your lung capacity. This will yield less breathlessness during the aerobic section of class. You may also begin to feel a little more flexible and stronger. Allow your body time to change, adjust, and improve. Before long you will see changes in your body that will reinforce your efforts.

What to Wear to Class

Comfortable clothes that provide ease of movement along with a good pair of aerobic or athletic shoes are all that you need. Generally, students wear leotards and tights, T-shirts and shorts, or warm-up suits. Cotton or a cotton-mix fabric provides the most comfort. Cotton "breathes" and helps your body maintain its normal temperature by pulling perspiration away from the skin. With warm-up suits, you perspire so much that you become too hot. If you do wear a warm-up suit, wear clothes underneath it so you can remove the top and/or bottom of the suit when you get too warm. Nylon, rubber, or nonpermeable clothes are not recommended because they trap heat and prevent the evaporation of perspiration.

Selecting Shoes

A good aerobic shoe not only feels good, but it also may help prevent injury. It is important to buy shoes that are lightweight and are supportive, can move with your foot, and can absorb shock. Shoes that do not absorb impact make you more susceptible to Achilles' tendinitis, shin splints, knee pain, and stress fractures.

The right midsole of the shoe can offset the stresses that may lead to injury. The most popular material used in the midsoles offers the best structure for absorbing shock. The material is ethylene vinyl acetate (EVA). The ability of the shoe's midsole to dampen the force of impact is measured in durometers. The higher the rating, the firmer the sole and the greater its shock-absorbing ability. The taller and heavier you are, the firmer the midsole needed.

When first selecting aerobic shoes, seek the advice of a knowledgeable shoe salesperson. Shoe manufacturers change designs frequently to meet market demands. A salesperson can best advise you on the advantages of one brand of aerobic shoe over another.

Types of aerobic shoes

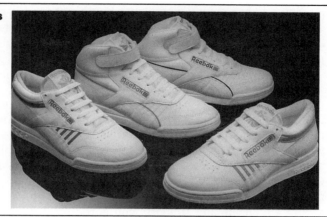

High- and low-cut aerobic shoes

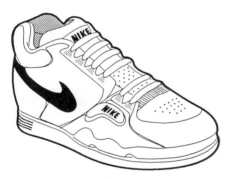

High-top aerobic shoe
Provides ankle support and
excellent cushioning.

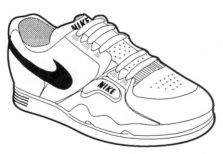

Low-cut aerobic shoe
Provides better flexibility
for all-around movement

Shoe diagram courtesy, NIKE products

Parts of a good aerobic shoe

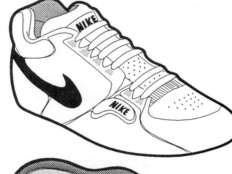

Upper
Flexibility and
comfort
are necessary
for workouts

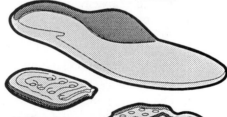

Sockliner
Provides
cushioning
and reduces
heat build-up
inside shoe

Heel cushion
Cushions and
protects the foot
from impact shock

**Forefoot
cushion**
Cushions the
metatarsal
heads from
impact shock

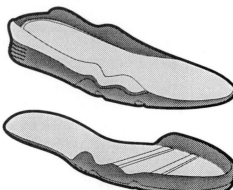

Midsole
Cups and
supports the
foot during
lateral
movement
and provides
arch support

Outsole
Made of abrasion-
resistant rubber,
with toe wrap

You need to decide whether to buy high-top, mid-cut, or low-cut shoes. The difference is individual. However, some people have weak ankles and choose the high- or mid-top shoe because it provides more ankle support. Other people prefer a low-cut aerobic shoe.

Some people put pads inside their shoes to add cushioning. Ask your shoe salesperson about pads or try them out yourself.

It is important to buy a shoe made for aerobic exercising. Some shoes now are called "cross trainer" shoes. These are designed for exercisers who regularly participate in running as well as aerobic dance exercise. Determine your needs, discuss them with a salesperson, and try out the shoe for as long as you can in the store. It is a mistake to just put on a shoe and buy it. Once the shoe is on, stand up, walk around, perform some of the movements you do in class, and decide whether you like the shoe. Trying on the shoe and seeing how it fits and supports you is the most important step in selecting the correct exercise shoe.

Summary

1. There are physiological, psychological, and social benefits from an aerobic dance exercise class.
2. To gain the benefits of an aerobics class, you must make exercise an integral part of your weekly routine.
3. Aerobic exercise provides the following physiological benefits:
   - The number of red blood cells increases.
   - The heart muscle strengthens and becomes more efficient as it pumps more blood with each stroke.
   - Lung capacity increases.
   - Bones become stronger and more dense.
   - The metabolic rate is elevated for several hours after exercise, thereby aiding in weight control.
   - Digestion and elimination are improved.
4. Psychological benefits also are a reward of aerobic dance exercise.
5. Following an aerobics class, people usually have a sense of well-being.
6. The components of a good class are warm-up, aerobics, strengthening and toning, cool-down, and flexibility.
7. Working out with adequate intensity three to five times per week yields cardiovascular fitness.
8. Improved fitness and changes in your physical appearance take time. Research indicates that it takes approximately eight weeks to experience increased efficiency in your cardiovascular system.
9. Remember, it is important physiologically and psychologically to allow yourself a 24- to 48-hour recovery each week.
10. Many people make the mistake of leaving class before they have completed a cool-down. Remember the two phases to a cool-down are:
    - to slowly return your heart rate to normal.
    - to stretch your muscles to prevent injury and stiffening.
11. Go to class physically, emotionally, and practically prepared to work out.
12. Wear permeable, comfortable clothes and supportive shoes. You don't need to be a fashion plate to participate in an aerobic dance exercise class!

CHAPTER 4

Your Personal Workout

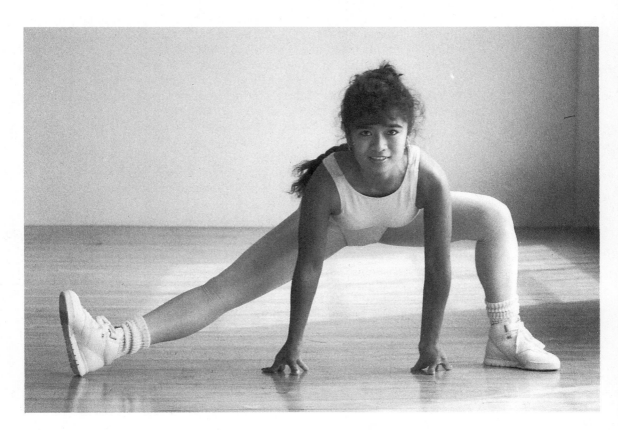

Outline

Your Pre-Class Warm-Up
Stretches and Isolations
    Head Isolations
    Shoulder Circles
    Rib Isolations
    Rib Circles
    Hip Isolations
    Hip Circles
    Deep Lunge
    Side Lunge
    Hamstring Stretch
    Quadricep Stretch
    Calf Stretches

    Ankle Circles
    Ankle Raises
    Heel Walking
    Sitting Straddle Side Stretch
Strengthening Exercises
    Push-Ups
    Reverse Push-Ups
    Abdominal Curl-Ups
    Donkey Leg Lifts
    Straight Leg Lifts
    Side Leg Lifts
Bent Side Leg Lifts
Pelvic Lifts/Buttocks Exercise
Checklist for Your Personal Workout
Summary

Once you have committed yourself to working out regularly, you must decide what you want to do for your weekly workout. Do you want to take an aerobics class four or five days per week? Or would you rather take a dance exercise class three times a week and walk and do strengthening and flexibility exercises at home two times a week? Whatever you decide, you must stick to it to gain the benefits of exercising.

As mentioned in Chapter 1, aerobic exercise is defined as exercise that utilizes oxygen for a sustained activity of two minutes or longer. Even though aerobic dance exercise classes and jogging are what come to mind when you think of aerobics, there are other forms of viable aerobic exercise. They are brisk walking, race walking, swimming, rapid bicycling, rebounder ("mini" trampoline) exercising, jumping rope, aqua aerobics, cross-country skiing, and rowing-machine work. All these activities are done alone, with the exception of walking and bicycling. Many people drop out of solo-type activities, whereas many enjoy the group aspect of an aerobic dance exercise class. Remember, you must enjoy the type of activity you select to be able to stick to it. Decide how you like to exercise, in a group or alone, and create a weekly routine for yourself. Exercising regularly must be as habitual as brushing your teeth. Your mind and body will become accustomed to exercising at a certain time on particular days and will miss it if you skip your regular routine.

Your Pre-Class Warm-Up

Remember, it is important to warm-up before you exercise to prepare your muscles and joints for a strenuous exercise bout. During the warm-up, you need to gradually raise your heart rate. Allow yourself eight to ten minutes for a good overall body warm-up. If you are taking an aerobic dance class, it is a good idea to gradually warm-up by walking around the class, stretching slowly and gently before class begins. Afterwards the following exercises would be good to do as part of your pre-class warm-up.

Stretches and Isolations

Caution: All head and neck exercises should be performed smoothly.

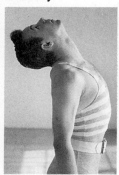

Head isolations
Lift your head up and down. Turn your head to the right and then the left. Repeat the set 4 to 8 times.

Caution: All head and neck exercises should be performed smoothly and in a relaxed manner. If you allow the neck to arch or roll back, you could put unnecessary tension on the cervical vertebrae.

Shoulder Circles
In a slow, smooth manner, circle your shoulders forward, up, back, and around 8 times. Then reverse the direction of the roll, and repeat it 8 times.

Head isolations

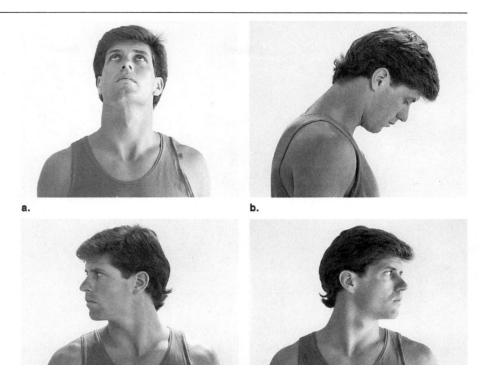

a.

b.

c.

d.

Shoulder circles

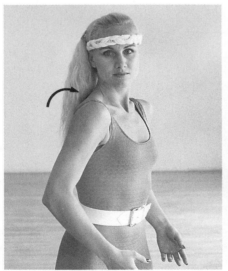

a.

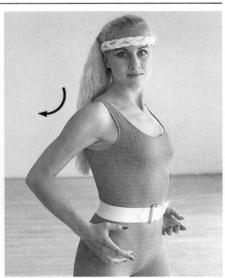

b.

Rib Isolations

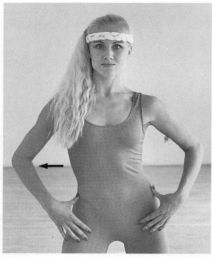
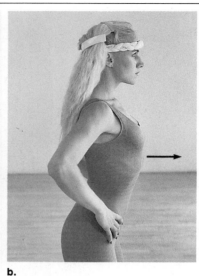

a.   b.

Rib Isolations

While standing with good posture, place your hands on your hips (this helps keep your hips from moving). Move your ribs forward, back to center, to the side, back to center, to the back, back to center, to the other side, and back to center. Repeat by reversing the direction of the rib isolations.

Rib Circles

Perform rib circles the same way as the rib isolations, but in a continuous manner. Do them several times in each direction.

Rib circles

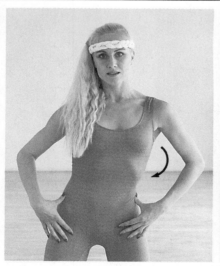
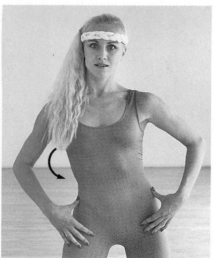

a.   b.

Hip Isolations

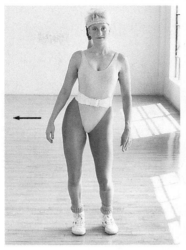 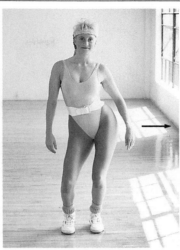

a.   b.

Hip Isolations

While standing with good posture, slightly bend your knees. Now smoothly tilt your pelvis forward and then backward. Repeat 8 times. Now, tilt your hips and pelvic area to the right and then the left. Repeat 8 times. Be sure to execute these movements in a smooth, sustained manner.

Hip Circles

While standing with good posture, slightly bend your knees. Smoothly circle your hips forward, to the side, to the back, and to the other side. Continue circling your hips at least 8 times. Now reverse the direction and perform the hip circles the same number of times. Keep your movements smooth and sustained. Jerking movements should be avoided.

Hip circles

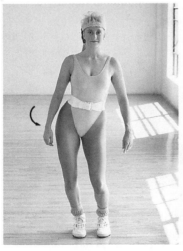 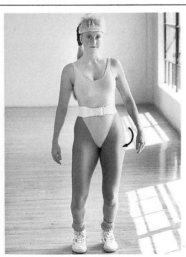

a.   b.

Deep lunge

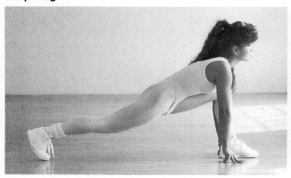
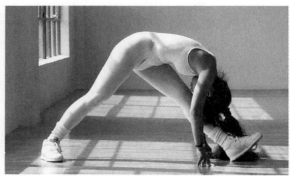

a.   b.

Deep Lunge

Begin in a standing position with good posture. With feet parallel, take a large step forward on one foot. Assume a deep lunge position, with hands on each side of your knee. The heel of your forward foot must remain on the floor, and the knee should be directly above the foot. Keep your extended back leg straight, with the toes of the foot pushing against the floor. Hold this position for 20 seconds. Now, straighten your forward bent leg and lift the toe up. Gently, without pulling, try to have your head touch your knee. This exercise will stretch your quadriceps, hamstrings, and the Achilles' tendon. Perform the exercise on your other leg. You may want to repeat the entire exercise for each leg.

Side lunge

Begin in a wide straddle position, with your legs and feet turned out. Bend one knee, and keep the other leg straight. Be sure to keep your knee over your toes and your feet flat while in the lunge position. Lift the toes of the straight leg, and let your hips sink as low as you can to get a nice stretch. Keep your hands on the floor for balance. Hold this position for 15 to 30 seconds, then perform it on the other side. Repeat the exercise on each side. This exercise stretches the muscles in the inside of your upper leg. These muscles are referred to as your hip flexor muscles.

Side lunge

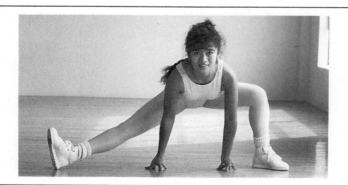

Hamstring stretch

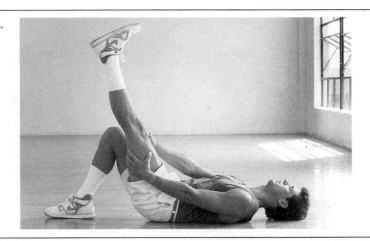

Hamstring Stretch

While lying on your back with your feet parallel, bend one leg and keep your foot on the ground for support. Lift your other leg up and try to keep the knee straight. Hold the lifted leg under the thigh for a minimum of 15 seconds, preferably for 30 to 60 seconds. This exercise stretches your hamstrings. Repeat on the other side. Perform another set.

Quadricep Stretch

Stand up with good posture. Keeping your supporting leg slightly bent, grasp your lower leg and gently pull your foot toward your buttocks. Proceed carefully, as this exercise can place stress on your knee joint?

Quadricep stretch

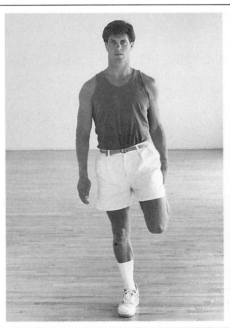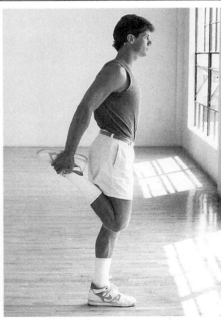

Calf stretches

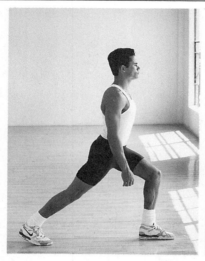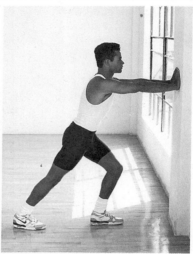

a.   b.

Calf Stretches
Perform either or both of the following calf exercises.

1. Perform a standing lunge by stepping forward with one foot so that your feet are approximately 1 to 2 feet apart. The front leg is bent, the back leg is straight with the toes facing forward. Hold this position for 20 seconds. Repeat on the other leg. Repeat the set again.
2. Stand facing a wall, approximately 2 feet away from it. Keep your body in a straight line and lunge forward, placing your hands on the wall about shoulder level. In the lunge position, your forward leg is bent, and your back leg is straight. You should feel a stretch in the calf of the straight leg. If you don't, adjust your position until you do. Repeat the exercise again.

Ankle Circles
While standing or sitting, circle your ankles 10 times in each direction. Repeat.

Ankle Raises
From a standing position in good posture, raise yourself up on the balls of your feet. Hold for 4 counts, and then lower yourself back to the floor in 4 counts. Repeat 10 times. Do another set, holding for 2 counts in each position.

Heel Walking
Lift your toes up and walk around the room on your heels. This strengthens your tibialis muscles.

Ankle circles while standing

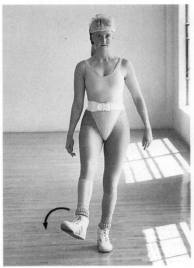

a.

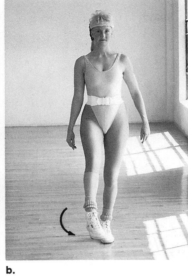

b.

Ankle circles while sitting

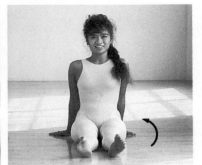

a.

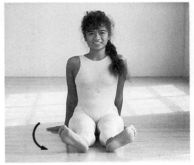

b.

Ankle raises

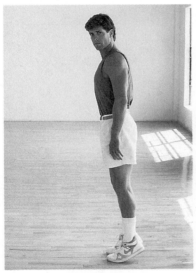

a.

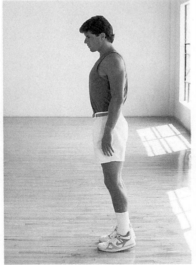

b.

Heel walking

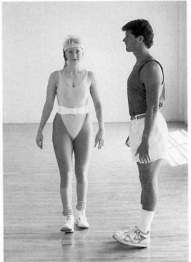

Sitting straddle side stretch

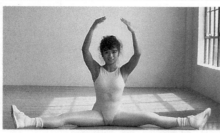

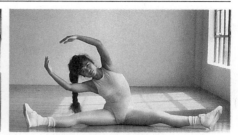

a.   b.

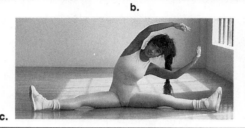

c.

Sitting Straddle Side Stretch

Sit on the floor in a wide straddle position, with your legs straight and your toes pointed. Hold your arms overhead, and stretch to the side. Hold this position for 10 seconds. Repeat on the other side. Repeat the total exercise several times.

    Variation 1: If your knee hurts, bend one leg so the foot faces the body as shown, and stretch over the extended leg. (See Photo).

    Variation 2: Instead of holding both arms overhead, stretch one arm overhead and the other one toward your toes, as shown in the illustration. (See photo).

**Variation 1:
Sitting straddle side stretch while bending one leg**

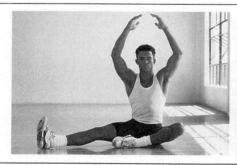
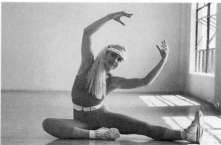

**Variation 2:
Sitting straddle side stretch**

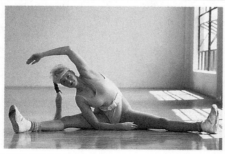
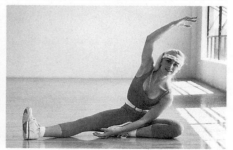

Sitting straddle forward stretch

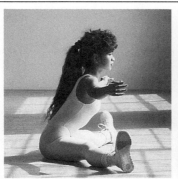

Side view

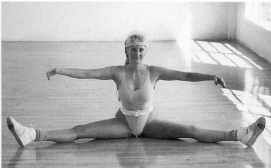

Front view

Sitting Straddle Forward Stretch

Sit on the floor in a wide straddle position. Let gravity pull your torso down, and lean your upper body forward. Be sure to bend from the hips. Hold this position for 10 seconds. Sit up, and repeat the exercise.

Strengthening Exercises

Push-Ups

Perform your maximum number of push-ups. Begin by lying on the floor face down with your fingers facing forward. Keep your feet together, your abdomen tight and pulled up, your weight on the balls of your feet and your body in a straight line. Push yourself up until your elbows are straight—but not hyperextended. Lower your body to the floor halfway (to the point of a 90° angle at the elbows) to perform one push-up. Repeat as many times as you can. This exercise will strengthen your shoulder girdle, pectoralis muscles, biceps, and triceps.

Note: Until you build up the upper body strength to perform full-length push-ups, you may need to perform knee push-ups. The upper body performance is the same as just described; however, the weight of the lower body is supported on the tops of the knee area.

Push-ups

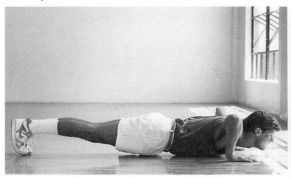

a.

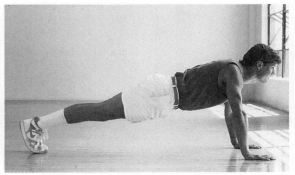

b.

Reverse push-ups

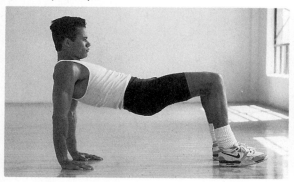 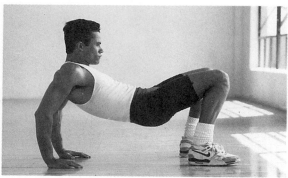

a.   b.

Reverse Push-Ups

This exercise strengthens your tricep muscles. Begin with your weight supported on you hands and feet and your back parallel to the floor. Your fingers must point toward your heels. Shift most of your weight toward your shoulders. Lower your body halfway to the floor, and then straighten your elbows to return to the starting position. Repeat as many times as possible.

Abdominal Curl-Ups

Lie on your back with your knees bent and your feet flat. Place your right hand across your chest and on your left shoulder and your left hand on your right shoulder. Lift your torso up halfway, keep your chin tucked toward your chest, and lift your head and shoulders off the floor. (If this hurts your neck, place your arms behind your head, touching opposite shoulders to cradle the head, keeping your eyes focused above you. Exhale, contract your abdominal muscles, and press your lower back to the floor as you curl up. Release the contraction. Lower yourself to the floor, being careful not to arch your back. Repeat the curl-up action as many times as you can.

Abdominal curl-ups

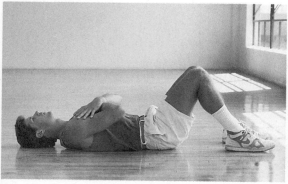 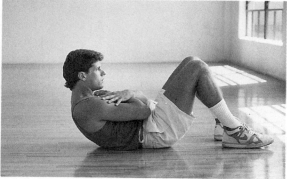

a.   b.

**Abdominal curl-ups,
front view**

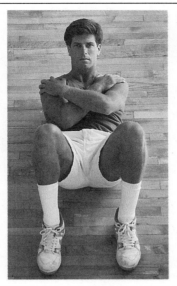

**Variation:
Abdominal curl-ups,
placing arms behind
the head**

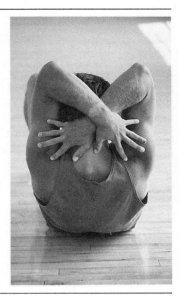

Donkey Leg Lifts

Begin on your hands and knees, with your weight supported on your forearms. Keep your head down. Be sure to pull your abdominal muscles in tight before you begin. Lift a bent leg up to hip level. Lift your leg in this position several inches, then lower it to hip level. Keep your hips parallel to the floor, and be sure you don't lean to one side. Repeat this exercise at least 20 times on each leg. This exercise strengthens your gluteal muscles in the buttocks.

Note: A variation of this exercise can be done while you are lying on your stomach (See photo on next page.).

Donkey leg lifts

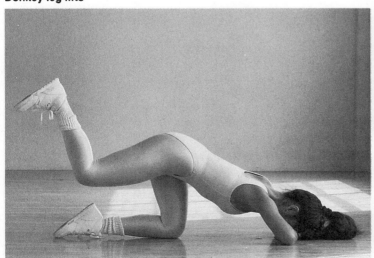

a.

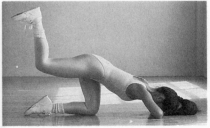

b.

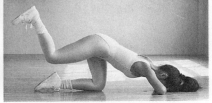

c.

Variation: Donkey leg lifts

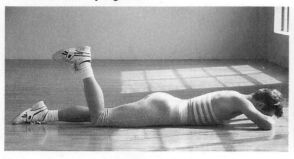 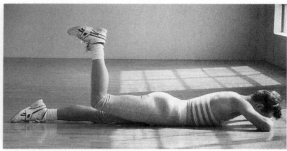

a.   b.

Straight Leg Lifts
Begin in the same position described for donkey leg lifts. Extend a straight leg directly in line with the shoulders to 3 to 6 inches below hip level. Now lift your leg up about 6 inches and lower it to the starting position. Never lift the leg above hip level, as that could cause stress on the lower back. Repeat this exercise about 20 times on each leg. Be sure you keep your weight evenly placed, and don't lean to one side. This exercise strengthens your hamstrings.

Straight leg lifts

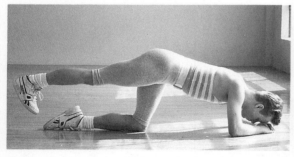 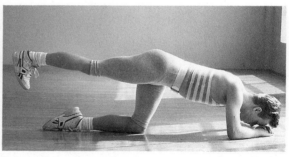

a.   b.

Side Leg Lifts
Begin by lying on your side. Have the arm closest to the floor support your head and have the top arm bent in front of your chest, with the palm on the floor. Lift the top leg straight up toward the ceiling, keeping it on a forward diagonal between 30°–45° from the body (See top view photo). Point the toe slightly towards the floor. Slowly lower the leg. This exercise works the abductor muscles located on the upper outside thigh. Repeat this exercise at least 20 times on each leg.

Side leg lifts

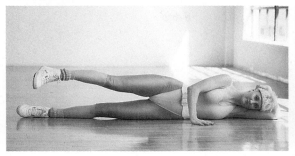

a.

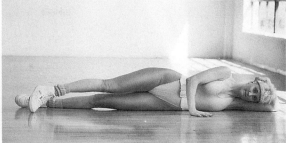

b.

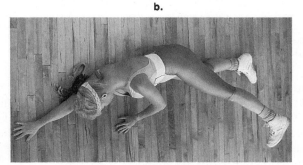

c. Top view

Bent side leg lifts

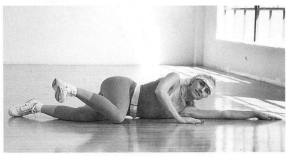

a.

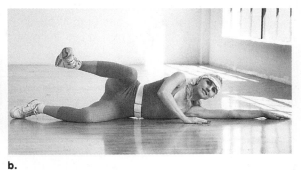

b.

Bent Side Leg Lifts

Begin by lying on your side. Bend both legs. Bring the top leg up towards the chest, and place the knee and lower leg on the floor for support. Lift the top leg up, hold it there, then slowly lower it to the floor. Repeat this 20 times on each side. This exercise strengthens the abductor muscles located on the inside of the thigh.

Caution: When performing the side leg lifts or the bent leg lifts, be sure to keep your back straight by contracting your abdominal muscles. In this way you avoid putting stress on your lower back.

Pelvic lifts/buttocks exercise

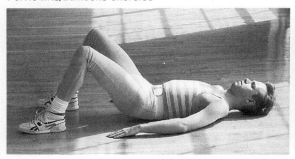 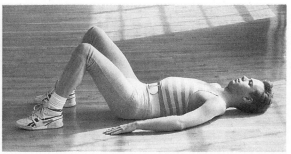

a.   b.

Pelvic Lifts/Buttocks Exercise

Lie on your back with your knees bent, the soles of your feet on the floor, and your hands by your sides. Keeping your lower back close to the floor, contract your abdominal muscles and your gluteal muscles to tilt and lift your pelvis approximately 1 to 2 inches toward the ceiling. Keeping your abdominal muscles contracted and your pelvis tilted up, smoothly contract your gluteal muscles. This contraction will gently lift your hips very slightly. Repeat approximately 20 to 30 times.

Caution: Do not lift the lower and middle back off the floor (See photo a.).

Variation: Turn your knees and feet out and continue the lifting motion just described another 20 to 30 times in this position. Return your knees to the parallel position. While keeping your pelvis firm and in the position described, bring your knees in toward each other and then out (See photo b.).

Variation: Pelvic lifts/ buttocks exercise

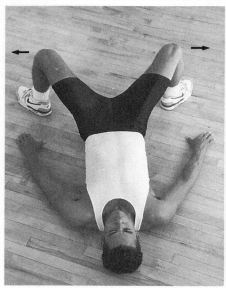 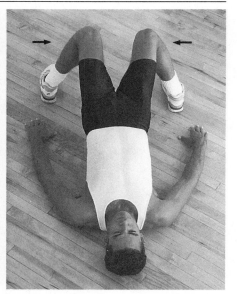

a.   b.

Checklist for Your Personal Workout

I plan to workout _____ times per week in an aerobic dance class and _____ times per week_____.

Directions: List the repetitions (REPS) and the date you do the following exercises.

Exercise	Date/Reps	Date/Reps	Date/Reps	Date/Reps
Head Isolations				
Shoulder Circles				
Rib Isolations				
Rib Circles				
Hip Isolations				
Hip Circles				
Deep Lunge				
Side Lunge				
Hamstring Stretch				
Quadricep Stretch				
Calf Stretches				
Ankle Circles				
Ankle Raises				
Heel Walking				
Sitting Straddle Side Stretch				
Sitting Straddle Forward Stretch				
Push-ups				
Reverse Push-ups				
Abdominal Curl-ups				
Donkey Leg Lifts				
Straight Leg Lifts				
Side Leg Lifts				
Bent Side Leg Lifts				
Pelvic Lifts/Buttocks Exercise				

Summary

1. You must commit yourself to a schedule for working out, or you may too easily find excuses why you can't exercise. Set a regular times to exercise in your weekly schedule. Once you are in the habit of working out, you will miss it when you can't exercise.
2. Remember, exercising is the best thing you can do for yourself!
3. Perform the exercises described in this chapter. Use the best possible body alignment to gain the most benefit from each exercise and to avoid injuries.

CHAPTER 5

Motivation: Identifying the Source

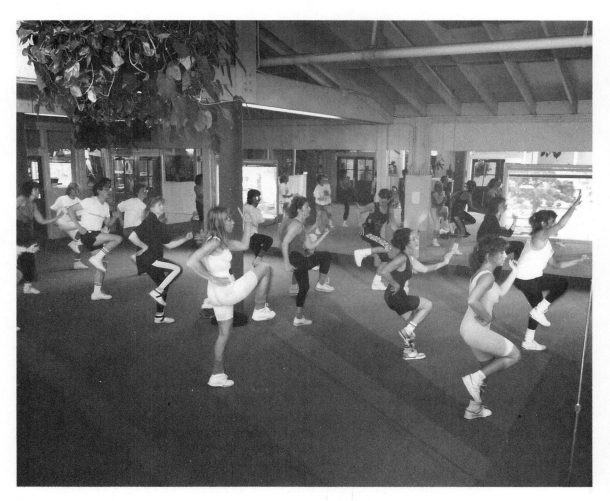

Outline

Negative Motivation
Positive Motivation
Inner Directed versus Outer Directed
Why You Keep Going
Mental Benefits of Aerobics

Setting Goals
Following the Goals with Action
Visualization
Checklist for Mental Imagery
Additional Motivation Tips
Summary

The desire to become physically fit through aerobic exercise is often evident when people begin a regular exercise program; however, the desire' may not be strong enough to sustain them through a long-term commitment. In order to stick with a program, exercisers can benefit from a variety of motivating tips and techniques.

Motivation refers to an inner drive that compels you to behave a certain way. You can be motivated to either pursue or avoid something. Aversion therapy is an example of training the mind and body to be repelled by a negative addiction such as smoking or alcohol. Incentive therapy refers to the rewarding of something pleasurable after the accomplishment of a certain positive behavior—for instance, receiving the keys to the family car for improving your grades.

This chapter contains some current thinking about motivation from the realm of the sport psychologist. It can be used to help you think about your own motivation as an aerobic exerciser.

Negative Motivation

The motivational technique that may have worked at one time for you will not necessarily motivate you several months down the road. Your attitudes and beliefs about what motivates you are in a constant state of change and adjustment. As you achieve certain short- and long-term goals, the elements of what spurred you on in the beginning no longer hold true at a later date.

The simplest way to identify your source of motivation is to identify and understand your particular needs. Here is an example. Steve is a 24-year-old computer programmer with a sedentary lifestyle and no great love of sports. He is gaining weight steadily and finds himself about 25 pounds overweight. He is surprised to discover that he can't climb the stairs to his apartment without being short of breath. The slightest activity seems to wear him out. As he takes a physical inventory, he realizes he is fast becoming as out of shape as his father, who died at the age of 43 from a heart attack. The fear of dying at such a young age scares Steve into signing up at a local health club. He dives feet first into a six-day-a-week jogging program, develops shin splints from doing too much too fast, and starts to grow discouraged that the weight isn't coming off as fast as he'd like.

The push behind Steve's desire to exercise arose from a negative source: fear of heart disease and death. Negative motivation isn't without its usefulness. It did get Steve started in the right direction. Many of us experience negative motivation in our everyday lives. For example, you go on a diet because you "can't stand this body anymore." An eight-year-old finally stops sucking her thumb because she is not going to let "those brats call me a baby anymore."

The negative motivation that drove Steve into exercising also drove him into an overuse syndrome, where he did not approach his fitness regimen with a realistic plan. A painful case of shin splints could keep Steve from exercising for several weeks—long enough to set up a cycle of despair, feelings of failure, complete inactivity, and more weight gain. Overcoming the obstacles to exercise may be more difficult the second time around for Steve.

The problem with negative motivation is that although it may be useful in the beginning, it is often not enough of an impetus to keep you going for a lifetime commitment. Negative motivation makes you run *from* something but not necessarily *to* anything. If the negative event or feeling that originally triggered the action starts to fade as a memory or grow distant in time, there will not be enough fuel to keep the wheels in motion.

Positive Motivation

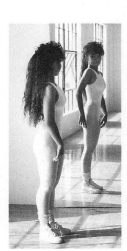

Positive motivation refers to attitudes, beliefs, and traits that spring from a source that enhances your performance, outlook, and confidence about exercise. Although it is more difficult to experience positive motivation in the initial stages of aerobic exercise, the nature of positive motivation is more sustaining in the long run. Here is an example.

Paula is a 20-year-old college senior who has devoted all her energy to studying and passing her final examinations. She admits to letting her body "fall apart," to surviving on junk food, very little sleep, and a complete lack of exercise. Now that she has to enter the career market, she wants to clean up her act, as she says, and get in shape for job interviews. As she starts taking aerobic classes three times a week, she finds they are tougher than she thought they would be. However, she is determined to achieve her goals of a five-pound weight loss in one month, a firmer physique in three months, and more energy.

Paula keeps a weekly log of the time, intensity, and frequency of her participation in aerobic classes, and also records her weight and activities each week. After three weeks, she is surprised to find that her eating patterns are starting to change. The desire to load up on high-fat, fast foods is starting to diminish. It's beginning to seem pointless to her to work so hard in exercise class, and then counteract all her good efforts with one quick fix of a greasy burger, fries, and milkshake. The aerobics class is becoming a little easier, but she remembers how tough it was in the beginning.

Paula is not alone. Sports psychologists have studied a transference of positive health habits to other lifestyle aspects among first-time exercisers. People who become committed to their exercise programs tend to cut down on smoking, eat a more nutritious diet, and reduce alcohol and substance abuse.

Positive motivation is self-reinforcing behavior that allows you to continue an action because of the rewarding benefits that slowly become evident. The human body was not made to be inactive, but rather, to be physically used. When we exercise regularly, the bones, muscles, heart, lungs, and blood vessels all begin to function better. If we do not stimulate our bodies into physical action, all of its functional capacities begin to decline at an accelerated rate. We begin to grow old before our time. When the benefits of regular exercise, both psychological and physical, begin to kick in—anywhere from three to twelve weeks after starting a program—positive motivation can take over the incentive job from the initial negative motivation. Positive or intrinsic motivation can last a lifetime.

Inner Directed versus Outer Directed

Have you ever known a person who is self-motivated? Self-motivated people are often the subjects of studies on exercise adherence. The personality traits that distinguish someone who is self-motivated are categorized and logged by researchers. One such trait is their ability to dismiss easily the types of excuses used by other individuals to not exercise—they don't look good that day, the class is too crowded, or they don't feel like going alone, for example. Self-motivated people are inner-directed; their goals come from an inner source instead of from others, such as family and friends.

Outer-directed individuals exercise because their boyfriend or girlfriend wants them to get in shape, because their friends joined a club, or because they want to please someone else. The chances of staying with an exercise program are less for the outer-directed than for the inner-directed person. Because there is no conscious awareness attached to the exercise, the outer-directed person does not always look forward to the benefits, and often drops out of the program before any real gains are made. It is possible for the outer-directed individual to shift to being an inner-directed exerciser. Think of someone you know who started exercising to attract someone's attention, but continued with the program regardless of whether the original motivator was still on the scene.

Why You Keep Going

What really keeps you going in an exercise program? What makes you lace up your aerobic shoes for one more class—even on days when you're dragging your heels? Research shows that for many people, the physical benefit of exercise is stimulus enough to keep them going. For others, the psychological benefits weigh more heavily. But for the majority, a sense of well-being and a positive glow following exercise tend to keep them positively addicted to their aerobic regimens.

Traditionally, exercise scientists have looked to the "runner's high" as a reason for long-term adherence. The "runner's high," reported by millions of aerobic enthusiasts, is a feeling of elation and uplifted spirits that lasts two to six hours after a vigorous exercise session. Physiologically, it follows from the release of a neurochemical transmitter, known as endorphin, which affects the body in a way similar to morphine. All sensation of pain or discomfort is masked, and a feeling of expansive self-worth occurs.

Today, some scientists are reporting that a psychological addiction to exercise kicks in with or without the release of endorphins, and that the positive mental attachment to the entire lifestyle of fitness is what keeps people coming back for more. In any case, the mental benefits of aerobics carry their own motivational message.

Mental Benefits of Aerobics

Research in the last two decades has led investigators to conclude that there are mental benefits of aerobics. These include:

1. Overall improvement in self-esteem.
2. Improved ability to cope with stress and tension.
3. Less free-floating anxiety.
4. Enhanced ability to concentrate and focus on one issue at a time.
5. Increased confidence about reaching goals.
6. Greater sense of self-acceptance.

7. Greater sense of satisfaction.
8. Overall improvement in mood.
9. Increased ability to relax.

Many of these mental benefits can enhance your physical performance during aerobics. The improvement in focus and concentration is a good example. By increasing the amount of resistance that you apply to contracting muscles during the floor work session of an aerobic class, you can actually increase the workload of that area, thereby increasing strength, muscular endurance, and total caloric burn. Another example of a mental benefit having an impact on performance is the ability to relax. Rest is an important part of physical training and can lay the groundwork for progression to the next level of goal achievement.

Setting Goals

The setting of goals and working toward their accomplishment is a significant part of all exercise programs, and aerobics is no exception. Goal setting also goes hand in hand with motivational techniques. The gratifying sense of achievement that follows when a goal is accomplished scores high marks as a motivational tool. The success can be transferred into all other areas of life that impact your exercise regimen, reinforcing the next wave of goals and efforts.

Goals for an aerobics program might include:

1. To gain both strength and cardiovascular endurance.
2. To develop more power.
3. To gain greater flexibility.
4. To lose excess fat.
5. To lower the resting heart rate.
6. To sleep more soundly owing to the right amount of physical fatigue.
7. To perfect a new choreography.

Following the Goals with Action

Motivation centers around the intensity and extent of your desire to accomplish a goal. The amount of enthusiasm you have in pursuing a goal indicates how much you really want to achieve that goal. Many people say they want to accomplish a goal, but only by looking at how fervently they pursue it can we accurately measure their desire for a positive outcome. In other words, talk is cheap. It's not enough to say "I want to get in shape." With aerobic exercise, the action versus the expression is what counts—it's what you do— not what you say.

Visualization

The practice of imagery or mental visualization is a technique that has been useful in motivating athletes to improve performance. The technique was pioneered by the sports coaches of the Eastern bloc nations and the U.S.S.R. and has been successfully employed by sports professionals and enthusiasts everywhere.

During mental visualization, the practitioner closes his eyes (usually) and envisions the actual performance of a sport or activity, with perfect execution, and a successful win or outcome. Greg Louganis, the U.S. Olympic champion diver, uses visualization to rehearse a dive, as does golf pro Jack Nicklaus.

As an aerobic exerciser, you can practice your routine mentally by seeing yourself performing the moves correctly. An advanced imagery technique allows you to move the action internally so that instead of closing your eyes and watching yourself do something, try to imagine others watching you flawlessly execute a perfect high-energy routine of a 60-minute class.

The technique of visualization works as a motivational tool because it helps you embrace the concept of yourself as a competent aerobic exerciser. Once you think of yourself as successful at something, you begin to adopt new attitudes and beliefs about yourself. This is part of the new "you." You can do this easily and with total enjoyment and have the ability to derive lifelong benefits from aerobics. Your motivation increases in proportion with your successful achievement of the task.

Checklist for Mental Imagery

1. See yourself from the outside as you practice a movement. Is your technique correct?
2. Feel your imaginary movement from the inside. Imagine yourself lasting the full 35 minutes of low-impact aerobics even when you're tired.

Additional Motivation Tips

Researchers have found that people who exercise at the same time every day are more likely to stick with an exercise program than people who vary their time. Another successful motivational technique is to find an exercise buddy. If the social context of exercise is friendly and inviting, the positive feelings are reinforcing. Finally, using a progress log and recognizing your achievement are highly motivational.

Summary

1. Try to identify a particular need for exercise. Look for something that can be solved or improved through regular exercise.
2. Beginning exercisers can be driven to launch a program because of negative motivation. Although useful, this is often not enough to lead them to a long-term commitment.
3. Positive motivation arises from the self-reinforcing benefits of exercise, both physical and psychological.

4. The inner-directed exerciser is someone who is self-motivated and overcomes common barriers to working out.
5. Outer-directed individuals may exercise because of someone else (or something else) in the early days, but can switch their source of motivation to inner-directed attitudes.
6. The psychological benefits of exercise coupled with the release of endorphins create a strong motivational force.
7. Setting and achieving goals for exercise can trigger feelings of success and self-worth throughout your life.
8. Visualization is a method of mentally rehearsing an ideal performance.

CHAPTER 6

Body Composition and Weight Control

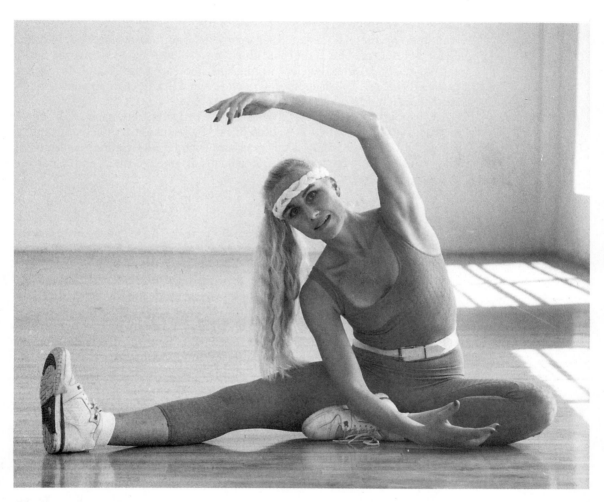

Outline

Basic Nutrition Guidelines
    Stick to Variety
    Carbohydrates
    Fiber
    Protein
    Fats
Checklist for Calories Contained in Four Food
    Groups

Water and Hydration
Vitamins and Minerals
Weight Control
Body Composition
Checklist for Calculating Desirable Body
    Weight
    Weight Loss
Summary

Basic Nutrition Guidelines

Your body requires a foundation of good nutrition to keep it running at its best. Proper nutrition can be accomplished through good judgment in obtaining the right amount of carbohydrates, proteins, fats, vitamins, minerals, fiber and water. Good nutrition is important not only in keeping you healthy, strong, and resistant to disease, but also in controlling your weight.

Stick To Variety

Hundreds of gimmicky eating plans come and go, but researchers find that eating a variety of foods is the most nutritious means of achieving overall health and longevity. A diet deficient in nutrients increases the risk of developing certain diseases. This is the best reason to avoid fad diets. Some can actually be dangerous.

A nutritious diet includes a wide variety of foods from each of the three caloric groups—carbohydrates, protein, and fat—including sufficient vitamins, minerals, fiber, and water. The American Dietetic Association recommends that your total daily calories be 30 percent fat, 15 percent protein, and 55 percent complex carbohydrates.

Carbohydrates

Carbohydrates, the primary energy source of the body, are of two kinds: simple and complex. Carbohydrates include starch, vegetables, fruit, and all forms of sugar. Complex carbohydrates (whole grains, pasta, legumes) serve as a long-acting fuel for the body. The American Dietetic Association and the National Institute of Health recommend that Americans increase their consumption of complex carbohydrates from the meager 25 percent that they've been eating to a level of 55 percent or higher. Carbohydrates provide only four calories per gram and are not as fattening as many people once believed. Carbohydrates are the exclusive fuel for brain function and are stored in the muscles as glycogen, which is used for short-term exercise. Carbohydrates are also "protein sparing," which means that when you consume adequate amounts of carbohydrates, your body is free to use dietary protein for tissue building and repair.

Carbohydrate sources are rich in nutrients, such as B vitamins and iron, as well as fiber. They also help promote a feeling of satiety or fullness. Sources of carbohydrates include milk, breads, cereals, legumes, fruit, and vegetables. Complex carbohydrates consist of a chain of simple sugars and can be recognized as "starchy" rather than sweet. Sugars, such as glucose and sucrose, are carbohydrates but are nutrient-poor and for the most part contribute empty calories. These are called simple carbohydrates. The average American consumes far too much of this simple sugar—almost 124 pounds of sugar per year, much of it hidden in processed foods.

Fiber

Fiber is obtained from whole grains, fruit, and vegetables. Fiber includes both the indigestible, crude type found in wheat bran and the water-soluble type found in beans and apples. It is important for promoting satiety, regulating bowel function, lowering cholesterol, regulating glucose absorption, and possibly reducing risk of certain bowel diseases. In general, Americans need to eat about twice as much fiber as they normally do.

Protein

Proteins are made of amino acids, the building blocks of tissues, enzymes, hormones, antibodies, and blood cells. Complete proteins (containing all the essential amino acids) are found in cheese, fish, chicken, milk, meat, and eggs. Vegetables and grains contain incomplete proteins, which can be combined with other types of foods to form complete proteins.

The recommended daily allowance (RDA) for protein is 1 gram of protein for every 2.2 pounds of body weight (.8 grams for every 1 kilogram). For a 130-pound woman, it is 44 grams; for a 154-pound man, it is 56 grams. The average American diet contains much more protein than necessary. Although protein contributes only 4 calories per gram, many foods that contain protein also contain fat and therefore can increase calorie consumption and contribute to the development of heart disease.

Fats

Fats are an important source of energy and warmth and are an essential part of cell structure. Some fats are essential for absorption of vitamins A, D, and E. These vitamins are also linked to the creation of blood lipids, steroids, cell membranes, and bile.

It is important to limit your intake of saturated fats and fats high in cholesterol, since elevated amounts in the bloodstream are associated with heart disease and stroke.

Fats, carbohydrates, and protein make up the caloric values of all foods. Proteins and carbohydrates each contain four calories per gram.

Fats are a calorie-dense food. One gram of fat contains nine calories. Therefore, fat-laden meals can add a tremendous amount of calories to your daily intake even though it may appear you are eating normal quantities of food.

A hamburger fried in grease, with oil-drenched french fries, and a saturated-fat milkshake together contain four times the calories of a meal consisting of fresh salad, applesauce, steamed vegetables, broiled fish, and iced tea with sugar. The typical American diet has too much fat, too many calories, and too few complex carbohydrates.

 Checklist for Calories Contained in Four Food Groups

---

1. Carbohydrates	4 calories per gram
2. Fat	9 calories per gram
3. Protein	4 calories per gram
4. Alcohol	7 calories per gram

Water and Hydration

The body generates heat during exercise, which must be dissipated through evaporation of sweat. Sweat is made up of water, sodium, potassium, and a few other trace elements. For those who participate in aerobic exercise classes, it is very important to replace the water. A good rule of thumb is to drink eight ounces of water for every hour of aerobics. If you're exercising in heat or high humidity, you'll need to drink more. Most dietitians agree that plain, cold water is the best beverage. Sports drinks, such as Gatorade, with added electrolytes are appropriate for strenuous exercise sessions that last over two hours, such as triathlons and marathons.

Vitamins and Minerals

If you are in good health and eat balanced meals from all four food groups (cereals and grain, meat, dairy, and fruits/vegetables), it's unlikely that you need to supplement your diet with vitamins and minerals. However, many nutritionists recommend a vitamin/mineral supplement if you tend to skip meals occasionally or not eat as well as you'd like. Megadoses are not necessary. Stay within the recommended daily allowances.

Vitamins and minerals are organic compounds that are not made by the body but are required for growth, maintenance, and repair of cells and tissues. For example, the B-complex vitamins help convert carbohydrate particles into energy molecules known as ATP. Vitamins C and E and the mineral iron are also important for sustaining good health in exercisers. As your exercise workload increases, adherence to a well-balanced diet grows increasingly important.

Weight Control

How to make proper food choices is the first lesson in weight management. But close on its heels, and gaining more impetus every day, is the importance of an increased level of physical activity as a lifelong tool for weight control.

Many factors influence a person's weight fluctuations. We used to think the simple mathematical formula of calorie intake versus calorie output was the chief determinant of body weight. Today, research shows us that the picture is much more complex. Heredity, set-point theory, brown fat deposits, altered basal metabolic rate, and other factors influence weight control. Heredity, for instance, is definitely gaining speed as a chief indicator of a child's future weight. In studies of identical twins who were raised apart and had very different eating patterns, the twins had similar excessive body fat deposits despite their dissimilar food intake and activity levels.

Set-point theory supports the notion that a body is genetically determined to remain at a certain weight, and that all efforts to increase or decrease that size are unsuccessful in the long run. Supporters of this theory point to the fact that metabolism automatically slows down whenever individuals diet, enabling the set-point weight to remain unchanged.

Brown fat versus yellow fat is another theory that supports a genetic predisposition to obesity. People of normal weight supposedly have more brown fat, a type of capillary-dense fat that surrounds and warms the vital organs and burns deposits of yellow fat as its chief fuel source. Obese individuals, as the theory goes, did not get their fair share of brown fat deposits at birth, and as a result, store yellow fat—the visible type that lies under the skin.

However, for those individuals close to their ideal weight, input/output still acts as an important energy equation. The theory can be summarized as follows:

1. Ingestion of calories exceeds expenditure of calories = weight gain.
2. Ingestion of calories is less than expenditure of calories = weight loss.
3. Ingestion of calories matches expenditure of calories = weight constant.

The problem with most weight-loss diets is that they concentrate on the wrong end of the energy equation. Simply decreasing caloric intake without increasing caloric expenditure usually does not result in permanent loss of fat.

You must expend and/or decrease calories by 500 to 1000 per day in order to lose one to two pounds per week. A loss of more than two pounds per week is most likely a loss of body fluid, not fat. It is interesting to note that 3,500 calories make up one pound of fat.

Rapid weight loss followed by periods of rapid weight gain is a common ailment among affluent Western societies. New evidence shows that this yo-yo effect induced by chronic fad dieting followed by a resumption of normal eating habits makes an individual fatter over the years. Your total body-fat percentage climbs with successive dieting, because the body grows alert to the "starvation" period while you're dieting and responds by lowering its metabolic rate. This is a survival mechanism, similar to the way hibernating animals store fat for the winter.

The goal of the dieter should be to heighten the body's basal metabolic rate (BMR) by consistent exercise, while maintaining sensible, well-balanced nutritional habits. The basal metabolic rate is the rate at which the body burns energy to conduct all the maintenance activities of daily life. BMR decreases with age and with decreased body surface area. It is slightly slower in women than in men. Exercise can help speed up the metabolic rate by increasing the amount of lean muscle in the body.

Body Composition

Body composition refers to the percentage of total body weight that is composed of lean body mass in relation to fat tissue. Body composition cannot be measured on a weight scale, but only through hydrastatic weighing (underwater), electrical impedance (measuring a current through the body), skinfold calipers (pinching subcutaneous layers), or circumferential measuring (of waist, thigh, and so on). Recommended amounts of fat for young men are 12 to 15 percent; for women, 18 to 22 percent.

The amount of fat on the body is determined by the number and size of the fat cells. The size of the cells can be stretched through overeating during any phase of a lifetime. One pound of fat stores about 3,500 calories in a form of liquid fat known as triglyceride. Another important fat in the body is cholesterol, which plays a vital role in heart disease, as discussed earlier in the text.

Checklist for Calculating Desirable Body Weight

To calculate desirable body weight:
1. Determine present weight. _____lbs.
2. Determine percentage of body fat, via skinfold or other method. _____%
3. Select the desired body fat. _____%
4. Subtract desired body fat from present body fat. _____%
5. Multiply the percentage of body fat to be lost by the present weight. _____lbs.
6. Leads to the desired weight. _____lbs.

Desired body weight equals lean body weight divided by percentage of lean body mass desired.

Weight Loss

To lose one pound per week, you should have a net deficit of 3,500 calories. This deficit is best created by expending more energy and limiting your daily caloric intake to 1,200 to 1,500, depending on your current weight, goal weight, and caloric expenditure. Use this formula to determine the number of calories you need to maintain ideal weight: For women, multiply your ideal weight by 16 if you are very active, 15 if you are somewhat active, and 14 if you are not very active. (For men, use 17, 16, and 15, respectively.)

For example, if you're a woman weighing 130 pounds and you are not very active, you need 130 x 14 = 1,820 calories a day. If you increase your activity by adding one hour of aerobics each day, you need 2,080 calories per day to maintain your weight because in the average aerobics class you burn 260 calories.

Summary

1. A well-balanced diet includes a wide variety of foods from each of the three caloric groups—carbohydrates, proteins, and fats—including sufficient vitamins, minerals, fiber, and water.
2. Research shows that the proportions of each group that Americans eat is not particularly healthful. The typical American diet has far too much fat and protein, and not enough complex carbohydrates.
3. The American Dietetic Association recommends that your total daily calories be 30 percent fat, 15 percent protein, and 55 percent complex carbohydrates.
4. Chronic dieting reduces the amount of lean muscle tissue in the body,

which has the net effect of gradually slowing down your metabolic engine.

5. Regular exercise adds muscle to the body and increases your fat-burning capacity.

6. The body is composed of both lean body mass and fat. The amount of fat on the body is measured by underwater weighing, electrical impedance, skinfold calipers, or circumferential measurements. The amount of fat recommended should not exceed 18 percent for men and should not exceed 22 percent for women.

CHAPTER 7

Injury Prevention

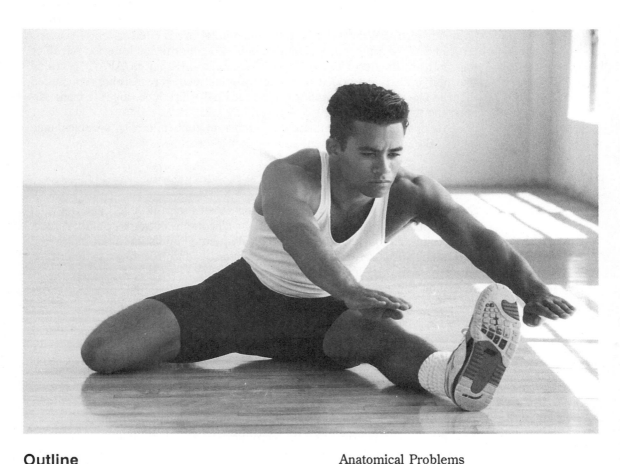

Outline

Prevention of Injury
Pain versus Exercise Discomfort
Treatment for Routine Injuries
Checklist for Treating Injuries
Overuse Injuries
    Plantar Fasciitis
    Achilles' Tendinitis
    Shin Splints
    Stress Reactions and Stress Fractures
    Knee Injuries
Common Causes of Aerobic Injuries
    Training Errors

Anatomical Problems
Improper Footwear
Training Surfaces
Program Imbalance
Use of Low Weights
Improper Body Alignment
Muscle Imbalance
Nonballistic Stretching
Exercises to Avoid
Heat and Humidity
Exercise-Induced Asthma
Exercise Intolerance
Cardiac Risk Factors
Summary

Prevention of Injury

Aerobic dance exercise has motivated a large segment of the American population toward personal fitness. It will continue to do so as long as the benefits far outweigh any potential for injury.

During the initial thrust of the aerobic dance movement, some early studies revealed injury reports as high as 75 percent for instructors and 45 percent for participants. Most of the injuries were the result of slow-to-heal, nagging overuse injuries, such as shin splints and tendinitis. In later studies, improper biomechanics and unsafe instructor techniques were cited as chief reasons for injury. The latest study, conducted in 1987 by the Institute for Aerobics Research and the Aerobics and Fitness Association of America (AFAA), revealed that injury rates had dropped to 35 percent for instructors; researchers concluded that the use of injury-prevention techniques helped reduce this rate from earlier reports of 75 percent.[1]

This chapter briefly outlines the significant contributors to aerobic-dance injury, along with recommendations for safe practice.

Pain versus Exercise Discomfort

Staying tuned to your body means being able to tell the difference between the pain of an acute or recent injury and the discomfort of exercise and overuse. Many injuries require immediate medical attention and should not be treated as routine. An injured ankle, for example, often needs to be x-rayed to determine whether there is a fracture.

Follow these simple guidelines to determine when to see a doctor. If you answer *yes* to any of the following questions, check with a physician.

1. Is the pain growing worse instead of better, despite rest and initial treatment?
2. Is mobility limited in the injured part?
3. Are you reluctant to place any weight on the limb?

Treatment for Routine Injuries

To treat routine injuries, use the acronym **RICE**, which stands for:

Rest
Ice
Compression
Elevation

Common sports injuries are usually successfully treated by following the four RICE steps. First, if you injure an area, rest. Do not exercise on it, or the problem will grow worse. You may move the injured part without placing weight on it in order to maintain circulation and promote healing to the area.

Second, apply ice on the injured part for 10 to 15 minutes at a time, as soon as possible after the injury. Slowly massage the area with an ice cube,

---

[1] *American Fitness*, Vol. 5, No. 8, 1987-8.

Checklist for Treating Injuries

Rest: Refrain from any further activity.
Ice: Apply ice massage for 10 to 15 minutes as soon as possible after injury.
Compression: Wrap affected area in elastic bandage.
Elevation: Keep the area above heart level if possible.

but protect the skin with a thin sheet. This constricts the blood vessels, reduces swelling, and numbs the area for a short while.

Next, securely wrap the area with an elastic bandage but not so tightly that you cut off all circulation. Following an ice massage, circulation increases. Compressing the injured area helps to prevent excessive swelling and further damage in the area.

Finally, elevate the injured area above heart level to prevent excessive swelling. This promotes healing as well.

Overuse Injuries

Overuse injuries result from repeated stress placed on the body as a result of too much activity too soon. Prevention is the best treatment, since overuse injuries are tough to completely heal. Excessive exercise causes a breakdown of cells in the muscles, tendons, bones, and cartilage. Damage to tissues causes swelling and pain. Pain usually convinces you to rest, which allows time for repair and growth of new cells. If you exercise despite painful warnings, further cell damage occurs, leading to tendinitis (inflammation of a tendon) and muscle strains. Stress reactions in the bones of the feet or the lower leg bones (tibia and fibula) can lead to tiny, painful stress fractures if the overuse continues unchecked.

Common Overuse Injuries

Plantar Fasciitis

Plantar fasciitis causes pain or burning on the sole of the foot, midfoot to heel. This injury occurs when the plantar fascia ligament, which connects the heel to the ball of the foot, is overstretched. Commonly called a sprained arch, this injury often results from a pronated (flattening of the arch) foot which pulls on the fascia or sheath covering the muscle.

Treatment often starts with a good arch support prescribed by a foot specialist (podiatrist). It is often necessary to apply an ice massage to the area after a workout.

Achilles' Tendinitis

This fairly common injury results in pain and stiffness in the heel cord, which connects the calf muscle to the heel bone. Wearing inadequate shoes, running on hard surfaces, doing improper warm-up, and doing insufficient stretching are some causes of Achilles' tendinitis.

Treatment consists of RICE (rest, ice, compression, and elevation), as described earlier in the chapter. Once healing has occurred, make sure you sufficiently stretch the tendon with a good calf stretch before and after your workout.

Shin Splints

This is a catch-all term describing any discomfort in the front lower leg, sometimes involving muscles and fascia, sometimes involving bone inflammation. Shin splints are fairly common among beginners, those exercising on concrete floors, or those without well-cushioned shoes.

Preventing shin splints is certainly preferable to treating them, since they tend to take several weeks or months to disappear. Exercise only on well-cushioned floors and wear good aerobic shoes. Also try to perform shin-strengthening exercises, such as lifting the toes toward the knee, with a weight wrapped around the forefoot. In cases of painful shin splints, RICE should give you relief.

Stress Reactions and Stress Fractures

Stress reactions or fractures may be confused with shin splints when they occur in the lower leg. Among aerobic enthusiasts, they are more commonly found in the feet. Stress reactions are a warning that the body is a victim of the overuse syndrome and that it's time to slow down, rest, and repair. Stress reactions that are ignored progress to full fractures.

Diagnosed by bone scan, stress fractures require medical treatment.

Knee Injuries

Knee injuries in aerobics are usually related to either (1) compression forces from jumping, resulting in a chronic ache, known as chrondomalacia; or (2) torque forces, resulting in a twisting of the knee, with injury to the ligaments or tendons. Proper alignment of the knees directly over the toes (never over-reaching them) is very important in preventing knee ligament strains.

RICE may help initially, but knees are very vulnerable to injury, so proceed with caution—knee injuries tend to make return visits. Check the soles of your shoes to make sure they are not overly worn. Try strengthening all the muscle groups that support and stabilize the knee. Working with an athletic trainer or physical therapist can improve the function and stability of your knees.

Common Causes of Aerobic Injuries

Training Errors

Doing too much too soon is a common training error. Suddenly increasing your training means that there is inadequate time for tissues to adapt to the challenging workload.

Do no more than 15 to 20 minutes of aerobics for the first few weeks, then advance to 30 minutes after two months. Advance gradually after that, as long as there are no signs of injury.

The beginner should take no more than six classes per week. The highly conditioned participant may safely take up to twelve classes per week.

Anatomical Problems

These include such things as one leg being longer than the other (which may throw off gait and alignment) knock-knees, fallen arches, rigid foot (very high arch), muscle imbalances, scoliosis or curved spine, pronated feet, and obesity.

Improper Footwear

Footwear is absolutely necessary in aerobic exercise classes to decrease the amount of shock transmitted up the body. The impact from footstrike can be two to three times greater without shock-absorbing shoes. Poor fitting or inappropriate shoes can also cause problems. Shoes that compact easily or lose their cushioning with use can cause stress injuries. Adequate lateral support in shoes is also very important in reducing the amount of shock.

Sometimes arch supports recommended by a sports podiatrist can reduce problems such as arch fatigue or excessive pronation (foot rolling to the inside).

Training Surfaces

High-impact aerobic exercise produces a percussive, vertical impact of footstrike, which leads to overuse injuries of the lower extremities. Impact is a product of force (how hard you work or how high you pick your feet up) times repetition.

The best types of floor surfaces are those which provide adequate cushioning yet maintain stability. Floors associated with the highest rates of injury include concrete, linoleum, and carpet over concrete. Optimal floors for aerobic dance are the following (see figure on page 66):

1. Suspended wood.
2. Coiled spring wood.
3. Shock-absorbing mats or special vinyl flooring.
4. Carpet over mats or rubber flooring.

Program Imbalance

Aerobic workouts that are not complemented with programs designed to improve flexibility, muscular endurance, muscular strength, coordination, agility, and balance can create an overall imbalance problem. Even periods of rest are considered essential to an exercise program. All of these factors are part of total fitness.

Use of Low Weights

Low weights can act as an added challenge for the cardiovascular and musculoskeletal systems once training gains start to plateau. But safe use of the weights is essential in order to avoid injury to the joints, tendons, and muscles. (See Chapter 8 for advice on the use of low weights.)

Standard floating wood floor

Dance flooring

5/8" plywood
finished one
side

2" x 4" wood strips
on end, 16" on
center

Foam blocks glued 6" on center to bottom of 2" x 4"

Portable floating wood subfloor
5 x 5" panels each
weighing about 50 pounds

Vinyl

Carpet

Interlocking
panel

Interlocking
panel

Foam blocks glued
6" on center

Foam blocks glued
6" on center

Dance flooring

Floor panels

Foam blocks

Improper Body Alignment

Proper body alignment during aerobic exercise can keep participants injury-free, with no back discomfort or knee pain. It is important to start with proper posture, which means keeping the planes of the body in a neutral midpoint. The trunk must be balanced in a neutral position, held in place by strong abdominal muscles in the front, and by strong gluteals, hamstrings, and lower back muscles posteriorly. The knees must be over the toes, with the weight forward on the metatarsals.

You risk fatiguing your muscles faster and injuring your joints if your body is not aligned correctly. Ankles, knees, hips, torso, shoulders, neck, and head—think of your body as a set of boxes to stack up.

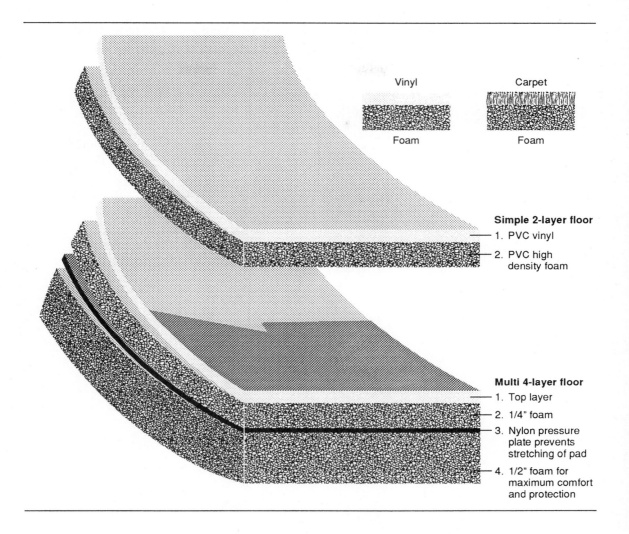

Vinyl

Foam

Carpet

Foam

Simple 2-layer floor
— 1. PVC vinyl
— 2. PVC high
    density foam

Multi 4-layer floor
— 1. Top layer
— 2. 1/4" foam
— 3. Nylon pressure
    plate prevents
    stretching of pad
— 4. 1/2" foam for
    maximum comfort
    and protection

When you stand, the patella (kneecap) and the toes should be facing the same direction. When lunging, keep the knees and toes in the same direction and make sure the knees never extend beyond the toes, laterally or medially.

Muscle Imbalance

Muscles oppose each other to move each of the body's levers at the joints. For example, the biceps contract, flexing the forearm while their opposing muscles, the triceps, relax and stretch. When the triceps contract, the forearm is extended, and this time, the biceps stretch. When muscles are out of balance or when one muscle is much stronger than its opposing muscle, injury is more likely to happen.

Muscle groups that come into play during aerobic dance include:

1. Adductors and abductors.
2. Quadriceps and hamstrings.
3. Gastrocnemius and tibialis anterior.
4. Abdominals and erector spinae.
5. Biceps and triceps.
6. Pectorals and rhomboids, trapezius.

Whenever a muscle or muscle group is strengthened, it should also be stretched. Otherwise, it will overpower its opposing muscle. For example,

Muscle groups, front view

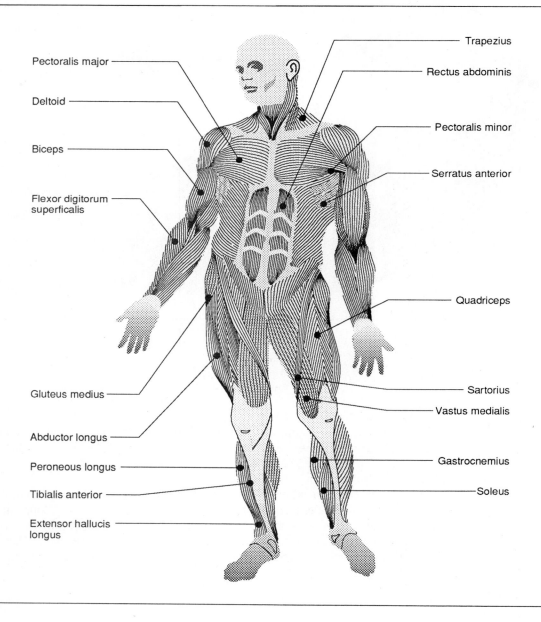

Pectoralis major

Deltoid

Biceps

Flexor digitorum superficalis

Gluteus medius

Abductor longus

Peroneous longus

Tibialis anterior

Extensor hallucis longus

Trapezius

Rectus abdominis

Pectoralis minor

Serratus anterior

Quadriceps

Sartorius

Vastus medialis

Gastrocnemius

Soleus

running can strengthen both quadriceps and hamstring muscles. If, after a run, an individual stretches the quadriceps but consistently fails to stretch the hamstrings, a serious imbalance occurs. The hamstring grows progressively tighter and shorter, pulling the pelvis out of alignment and creating low back discomfort. Of course, stretching alone does not prevent serious strength imbalances. Attention should also be paid to balancing the strength training regimen. However, it is important that opposing muscle groups be stretched to the point of mild tension and held for a minimum of 20 seconds during cooldown.

Muscle groups, back view

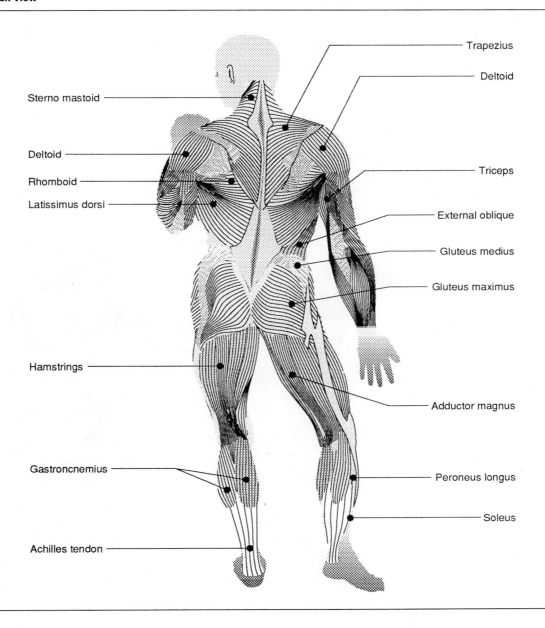

Trapezius

Deltoid

Sterno mastoid

Deltoid

Rhomboid

Latissimus dorsi

Triceps

External oblique

Gluteus medius

Gluteus maximus

Hamstrings

Adductor magnus

Gastroncnemius

Peroneus longus

Soleus

Achilles tendon

Nonballistic Stretching

Ballistic stretching is not recommended during warm-up or cool-down. As discussed earlier, ballistic or bouncing stretch is one that elicits the stretch reflex, a protective reflex of the neuromuscular system, similar to a knee jerk. It prevents the muscle from overstretching by actually contracting it. Some exercise professionals believe that static, slow stretches (nonballistic) elongate the muscle, helping to rid the fibers of toxic by-products of metabolism such as lactic acid. Stretch to the point of mild tension, not pain. Go only as far as you can tolerate comfortably.

Exercises to Avoid

The following exercises place undue stress on the joints, seriously overstretch ligaments, and create torque-like or twisting forces to vertebrae and joints throughout the body.

1. Back arching or hyper-extension.
2. Hurdler's stretch.
3. Yoga plough.
4. Straight leg lifts.
5. Windmill toe touches.
6. Deep knee bends.
7. Full sit-ups.
8. Rapid side to side twisting.
9. Side leg swings on hands and knees.

**Exercises to avoid:
Back arching or hyper-extension**

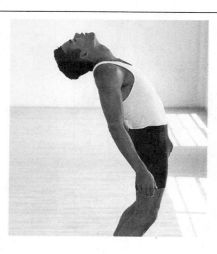

Hurdler's stretch

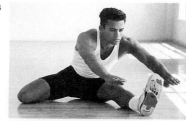

a.

Top view

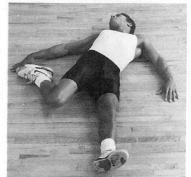

b.

Yoga plough

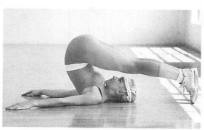

**Exercise to avoid:
Straight leg lifts**

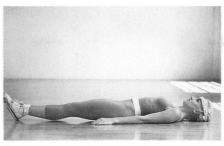

a.

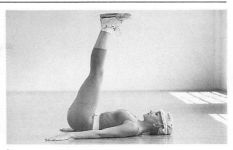

b.

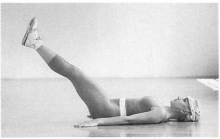

c.

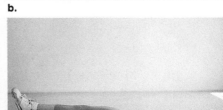

d.

Exercises to avoid: Windmill toe touches

Deep knee bends

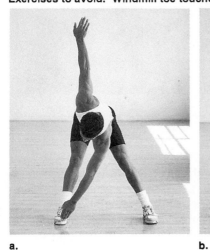

a.

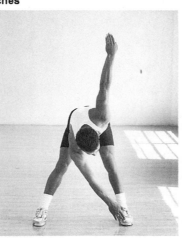

b.

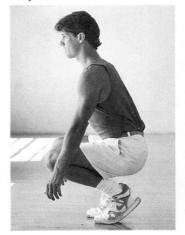

Full sit-ups

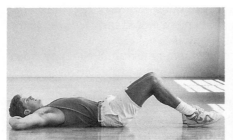

a.

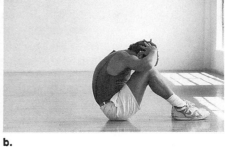

b.

**Exercise to avoid:
Rapid side to side
twisting**

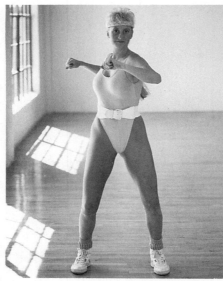

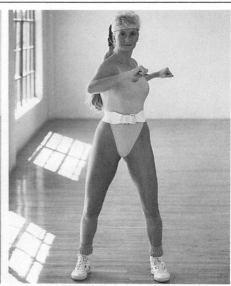

a.   b.

**Side leg swings on
hands and knees**

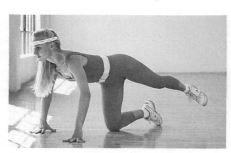

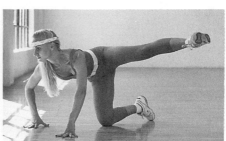

a.   b.

Heat and Humidity

A major by-product of muscular work is heat, which raises the body's core temperature. The circulating blood carries this heat to the surface of the skin, where it is released via the opening of pores and the evaporation of sweat. The sweat produced during one to two hours of exercise consists primarily of water, along with some minor amounts of sodium, urea, uric acid, and amino acids.

Drinking 8 ounces of water for every 20 minutes of exercise is a good rule of thumb for rehydration. Water is the chief regulatory element for keeping your body's aerobic engine cool.

Never exercise in clothing that inhibits evaporation of sweat from the body (materials such as nylon and nonpermeable plastic wraps); otherwise, serious heat injury can result.

On hot and humid days, sweat may not have a chance to evaporate, causing the body to retain heat and raise your core temperature. Lower the intensity of exercise during these periods so that heat injury is not risked.

Exercise-Induced Asthma

This is a type of allergic response to exercise characterized by wheezing and difficulty in breathing. Inhalant medication can alleviate the symptoms. Check with a physician before proceeding with exercise should these symptoms arise.

Exercise Intolerance

If you have any of the following abnormal responses to exercise, you need to check with a physician before continuing the exercise program. These symptoms could indicate cardiovascular disease or an impending heart attack or stroke.

1. Light-headedness.
2. Dizziness.
3. Ringing in ears.
4. Excessive shortness of breath.
5. Chest pain, heaviness, or burning.
6. Jaw pain.
7. Arm pain, numbness, or tingling.
8. Nausea or vomiting.
9. Irregular pulse or sudden palpitations.
10. Fever.
11. Hives, swelling, or itching.
12. Severe aches and pains in a particular area of the body.

If any of the above conditions develop while exercising, stop immediately, cool down if possible, and seek medical attention.

Cardiac Risk Factors

If you have a history of cardiovascular disease, always seek medical clearance before starting an exercise program. The following list of risk factors contribute to the incidence of heart disease.

Advanced age: Risk increases over age 50.
Male gender: Risk is higher in males than in females.
High blood pressure: A chief contributor of heart attacks. Upper limit for young adult is 140/90; lower limit is 70/50. Normal range is around 120/80.
Family history of heart problems: Positive history means frequent checkups.
Sedentary: Inactivity increases cholesterol and contributes to obesity.
Smoker: Increases the risk of heart disease fourfold.
Diabetic: Risk is greater for insulin-dependent diabetes.
Elevated cholesterol and trigylceride levels in the blood: Contribute to heart disease and stroke.

If you have a history of any medical condition, you should get medical clearance before engaging in vigorous aerobic exercise. Exercise can be an excellent therapeutic tool in the treatment of diabetes, obesity, cardiovascular disease, stress disorders, and musculoskeletal limitations, when supervised properly.

Summary

1. The most common types of injuries in aerobic dance are known as overuse injuries, which result from too much stress over too short a period. Cellular damage to muscles, bones, and other tissues requires time for repair and growth of new cells. Exercising despite painful warnings can lead to further damage.
2. A standard initial treatment for minor sports injuries consists of rest, ice, compression, and elevation, commonly called RICE. Ice should be applied to the injured part for at least 10 to 15 minutes, followed by a secure wrap and elevation.
3. Common overuse injuries include inflammation of the sole of the foot (plantar fasciitis) and the Achilles' tendon, shin splints, stress reactions and fractures, and knee injuries.
4. Attention should be paid to balancing overall fitness with programs for flexibility, muscular endurance, strength, coordination, agility, and balance. Opposing muscles should be balanced in strength and flexibility so that injuries and tears are avoided.
5. Proper body alignment during aerobic exercise is an essential component of injury prevention.
6. Certain movements should be avoided altogether in a safe aerobics program. These include ballistic or bouncing stretches during warm-up and cool-down, and any exercises that place undue stress on the joints or ligaments.
7. An aerobic exercise enthusiast should be in tune with his or her body and learn to recognize any sign of exercise intolerance, such as overheating, difficulty in breathing, light-headedness, or pain.
8. Anyone with a history of medical problems or physical limitations should seek physician approval before beginning a vigorous aerobic program.

CHAPTER 8

Low-Impact Aerobics

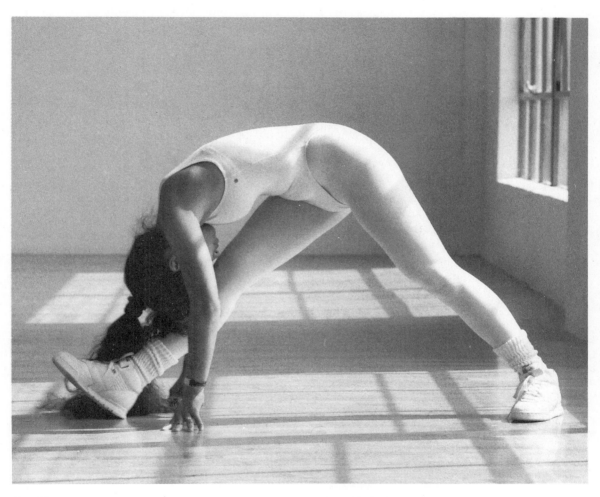

Outline

Definition
Impact and Injuries
Protecting the Knees
Checklist for Knee Protection
Low-Back Precautions

The Question of Weights
Low Impact versus Low Intensity
Aqua Exercise
Benefits
Summary

Definition

Low-impact aerobics (LIA) is a relatively new form of aerobic exercise that is perfect for anyone who wants to avoid the jumping and jarring movements performed in traditional high-impact classes. The basic rule is to keep one foot on the floor at all times while performing vigorous upper body moves. There is, however, a lot more to low impact than simply "grounding" a high-impact class. Instructors must try to make their students mentally alert as to how their bodies are moving. They not only have to concentrate on intensity of a movement, but they also have to focus on a full range of motion and smooth transitions. The careful patterning and sequencing of a class are instrumental in achieving the desired cardiovascular training effects.

Some experts say that low impact is not so much a new trend as it is simply a new name. Those who have conducted classes for over fifteen years find it interesting to watch the return of dance like movements, which are replacing the jumping and hopping of traditional aerobics.

The following guidelines should help make a low-impact class safe, yet enjoyable.

Impact and Injuries

Whenever the feet come into contact with the floor, there is an impact. Frequent, high-impact movements that are not done safely may lead to injuries. Injuries from high-impact aerobics are generally overuse injuries relating to compression or impact trauma. As discussed in the previous chapter, they include shin splints, stress reactions, stress fractures, plantar fasciitis, tendinitis, and so on. Low-impact aerobics emerged with the goal of reducing the impact of jumping and running-in-place movements.

Low-impact aerobics stresses vigorous upper body movement, while focusing on smooth transitions and intensity of movement.

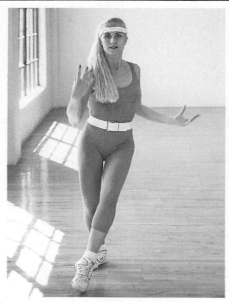 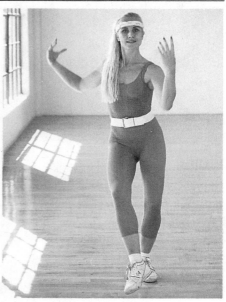

a.   b.

Has the injury rate actually decreased? It's likely that injuries to the lower extremities have decreased, but more research is needed to prove it. It is also likely that the sites of injuries have shifted from shins, Achilles' tendons and feet in high-impact aerobics to knees, lower backs, shoulders, and arms in low impact. Before any definite conclusions can be made regarding the safety of low-impact aerobics, research needs to be done.

As in high-impact classes, in low-impact aerobics you need to pay attention to proper footwear and resilient floor surfaces. Floors should be either carpet over mats, highly stable mats, or spring or suspension wood floors. Shoes, once again, are important. The quick side-to-side movements you make during low-impact aerobics require extensive lateral support in an aerobic shoe.

However, when all factors are taken into account, the instructor's technique seems to be the single most important consideration in injury prevention. The best pair of aerobic shoes and the latest, safest floor won't protect you from improper biomechanical (body position) form, or dangerous exercises.

Protecting the Knees

The quick, lateral movements in a low-impact class can endanger the knees. Be aware of your center of gravity (in the center of your hips), and keep it balanced over the midfoot. Make sure the knees never overshoot the toes when you do side lunges. This action overstretches knee ligaments and makes the joint unstable. Keep your knees facing the same direction as the lower leg and toes when you do side lunges. Whenever the knee points in one direction and the leg twists in the opposite direction, a force known as torque creates excessive stress on the knee joint. Be sure to pick your feet up— don't let the toes drag against the floor—when switching direction.

Also, try to build the strength in your quadriceps (front thigh muscles) and hamstrings for added protection. Don't expect your knees to compensate for weak leg muscles.

Checklist for Knee Protection

1. When standing, never overextend the knees beyond the toes.
2. Make sure the knee, ankle, and midfoot are in straight alignment.
3. Never bring the hips below the level of the knees in a working squat or lunge.

Low-Back Precautions

Make sure you don't arch your back when you raise your arms overhead, and don't lean forward without supporting your upper body weight. Slow down the movements and avoid hyperextending the shoulder joint. When standing, the best way to avoid arching the back is to make sure your abdominal muscles are contracted, pelvis is tucked, rib cage is lifted, and knees are slightly bent.

Instructors learn the proper use of weights in low-impact aerobics

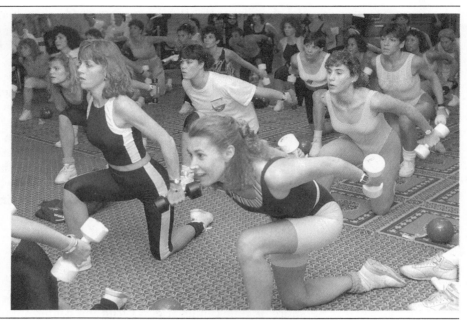

The Question of Weights

You may want to try using hand-held or wrist weights in class. Some instructors feel that weights give an added boost to the cardiovascular challenge in a class once individuals have reached such a high level of conditioning that it's difficult for them to attain their target heart rate. However, research indicates that weights under two pounds do not significantly contribute to the cardiovascular conditioning effect. If your arms are lacking any muscular definition or tone, weights may put you on the road to minor gains in muscular endurance and strength. On the whole, most instructors have a policy of using weights during the conditioning portion of a class but never during the aerobics portion. In so doing, they are consistent with the AFAA Standards and Guidelines for Low Weight/Low-Impact Aerobics.

Keep the movements controlled, smooth, and within the normal range of motion for the joint. Rapid jerking movements with weights can cause problems in the elbow joint, forearms, shoulders, and arm muscles. Again, make sure you are not hyperextending or bending the joint past its normal anatomical position. Also, don't snap the joint. Tendons in the wrist and forearms can be inflamed due to overuse of weak muscles and overgripping of low weights. Don't let the arm snap up and roll backward. The head of the bicep muscle can become seriously inflamed, requiring about four to six weeks of rest, plus physical therapy and medical treatment.

Weights are for nonbeginners only. People who can perform sixteen repetitions without fatigue are probably ready for weights. Start with the smallest weight (one pound), then progress gradually but do not exceed three pounds during aerobic work. Ankle weights should be used only during strengthening exercises for the lower body—never during aerobics. Remember to keep weights off during the warm-up and cool-down portions of class.

Joints, tendons, and muscles need at least a ten-minute warm-up period to prepare for the added stress of weights.

Beginners tend to grip the hand weights too tightly and actually impair blood flow in the arms owing to a continuous isometric contraction. This action can raise blood pressure to serious levels. People with high blood pressure or a history of stroke or heart disease should consult their physicians prior to exercising with weights. If joint soreness or muscular pain develops, stop using weights and rest.

Let your heart rate monitor whether you should add or subtract weights. Your heart rate will climb whenever additional weight is added.

Low Impact versus Low Intensity

Low-impact often gets confused with low intensity. Low-impact refers to a reduced impact stress on the feet, legs, knees, and hips—not to a lower intensity. Low intensity refers to a reduced workload, or working at a lower heart rate. There are beginner, intermediate, and advanced classes for people at various levels of fitness.

Lower the intensity of a low-impact class by keeping arm movements below shoulder height until you gradually gain strength. Instead of performing high-stepping movements, simply march in place. Don't raise the knees quite as high. Avoid complex patterns if you're a beginner. You'll be ready to join in again if you can carry on a brief conversation comfortably, or if you remain at your target heart rate while working.

Aqua Exercise

According to the Aquatic Exercise Association (AEA), water aerobics is a relative newcomer to the fitness scene. It is gaining popularity because of its nonstressful, nonpercussive style. Jane Katz, Ed.D., author of the *W.E.T. Workout*, advocates water aerobics for overweight individuals. The buoyancy and resistance of water make a 150-pound person weigh only 15 pounds. Water aerobics is usually done in chest-deep water; swimming is not usually part of the routine. Classes are geared to all types of people: rehabilitating athletes, seniors, pregnant women, arthritis patients, and people who simply love the water. For more information on water aerobics, contact AEA, P.O. Box 497, Port Washington, WI 53074.

Benefits

The benefits of a low-impact class are identical to those of any aerobic exercise training program. The benefits include:
1. Lowered resting heart rate.
2. Lowered resting blood pressure.
3. Reduced triglycerides.
4. Increased HDL cholesterol (the protective type of cholesterol).
5. Enhanced basal metabolic rate.
6. Less overall body fat.
7. Improved cardiopulmonary efficiency.
8. Improved ability to cope with stress.
9. Preferred form of aerobics after returning from an injury.

However, just like with traditional aerobics, you achieve benefits only if you exercise with sufficient frequency, duration, and intensity. The aerobic portion of class must be at least 20 minutes long, with heart rates in the training heart rate range, and you must attend class (or get the equivalent workout outside of class) at least three or four times per week.

It is premature to state whether there will be less injuries in low-impact aerobics compared with traditional aerobics. We may just see a shift in injuries from shins and feet to shoulders and backs. Any part of the body can be subjected to overuse injuries. Injury is usually a sign of too much, too soon. Compression or impact trauma is not the only cause of overuse injuries. Therefore, use common sense to pace yourself.

Summary

1. Low impact can be an enjoyable form of exercise and a welcome change from high-impact classes.
2. Low-impact aerobics is a relative newcomer to the aerobic field, and is welcomed by those who wish to avoid the jumping in a high-impact class. It consists of vigorous upper body moves coupled with leg movements that allow you to keep one foot on the floor at all times.
3. It is important to protect the knees when performing the quick lateral movements in a low-impact class. Try to avoid extending the knee beyond the toes. Also try to keep the knee and the foot pointing in the same direction whenever switching back and forth quickly.
4. Hand-held weights can add a challenge to the cardiovascular system for advanced exercisers. Some precautions should be taken when working with weights. Make sure your back does not arch when your arms are raised overhead, and definitely avoid rapid, jerking movements. Work the weights with a slow, controlled style.

CHAPTER 9

Pregnancy and Dance Exercise

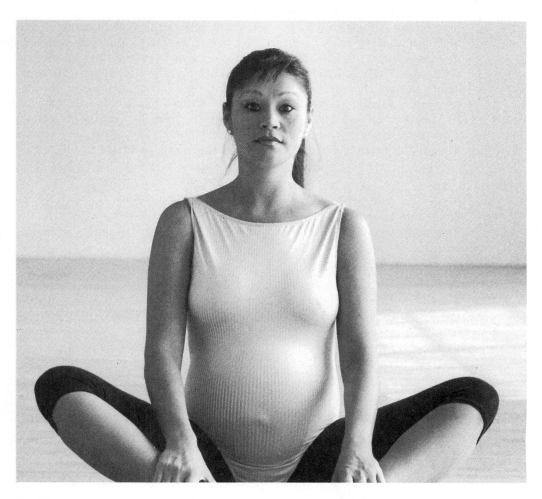

Outline

Value
Special Precautions
Modifications of an Aerobic Exercise Program
    Cardiovascular Work
    Floor Work
    Cool-Down Stretches
Special Exercises
    Low-Impact Movement
    Kegels

Standing Work
Controversial Exercises
Exercises to Avoid
    High Knee Lifts
    Quick Lateral Movements
    High-Impact Jumping and Jarring
    Weights
    Traditional Rejects
    Prone Position
Summary

Value

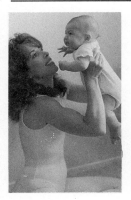

Pregnancy and aerobic dance exercise can be safe partners. Aerobic dance can have a healthy and positive effect on a mom-to-be, and help her with a rapid recovery during the post-partum period. A prenatal class should be taught by a trained professional to meet the physical and emotional needs of the pregnant exerciser. Classes offered in conjunction with childbirth education are among the most conscientious programs.

Exercise does not necessarily decrease labor time or insure a healthier baby. It does provide quite a few benefits directly to the mother, and indirectly to the developing fetus. Research supports the finding that the exercising mother-to-be can maintain her own cardiovascular fitness, musculoskeletal strength, and flexibility. Benefits to the fetus are less well defined. However, sufficient data support the finding that the fetus is not endangered during a pregnant woman's consistent exercise for periods of 15 minutes or less when her heart rate is no higher than 140 beats per minute. As the pregnancy advances, the woman and her physician should continue to evaluate her tolerance to aerobic exercise, and whether or not she should exercise to full term.

Special Precautions

Medical Clearance
Pregnant women should seek physician clearance before beginning or altering an exercise program.

Fluids
Pregnant women should be encouraged to drink freely before, during, and after a workout to avoid dehydration. Exercise can raise the body's core temperature to dangerous levels that risk fetal health, especially during the first three months of pregnancy.

Modifications of an Aerobic Exercise Program

Important modifications of the traditional aerobics class need to be made for pregnant women. The following is a list of general modifications and guidelines adapted from both the American College of Obstetricians and Gynecologists (ACOG) and a symposium, lecture and video course called *Pregnancy the Aerobic Way*, developed by Bonnie Rote, RN and AFAA consultant, and Kenneth Sekine, MD.

Warm-Up
The warm-up should be longer than in regular classes, due to the pregnant woman's increased risk of orthopedic injury. Ten to twelve minutes is the minimum time period for warm-up. During pregnancy, estrogen and progesterone cause tissues and joints to soften and become unstable. When joints are unstable, ligaments and tendons are in greater danger of tears or strains. The enlarged breasts and uterus alter the center of gravity and produce a greater strain on the lower back. An increased load is also placed on the sacroiliac and hip joints, which can feel like a sore tailbone at times.

Altered body alignment: Pregnant versus non-pregnant

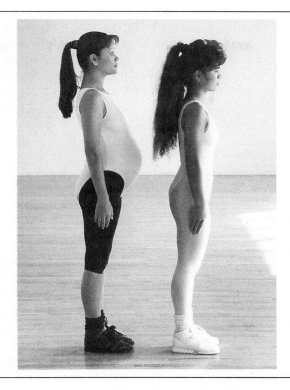

It is fatiguing for pregnant exercisers to maintain proper body alignment while standing; therefore, many thoughtful teachers have developed methods of warming up while on the floor. Smooth, controlled, static stretches are essential to a proper warm-up. Static stretches for the hamstring, inner thigh, and calf can all be performed on the floor. Ballistic movements should never be performed during warm-up or cool-down.

Rhythmic limbering is the second essential element to a proper warm-up. Mild walking and rhythmic upper body movement are both good warm-up exercises.

Cardiovascular Work

During pregnancy, the mother's blood volume increases by 50 percent. This dilute volume results in a lower oxygen-carrying capacity, which reduces the cardiac reserve during physical activity. In addition, the expanding uterus reduces the size of the lung cavity, causing a mild hyperventilation during rest that does not increase proportionately with exercise. Overall, this means that many pregnant women may be unable to maintain high levels of aerobic activity.

To adapt to aerobic work when pregnant, lower the target heart rate to 60 percent of maximum for beginners, gradually increasing to 70 percent of maximum for intermediate to advanced. It's wise to maintain a target heart rate of 65 percent during the final stages of pregnancy. The American College of Obstetricians and Gynecologists recommends never exceeding 140 beats per minute (see target heart rate calculations).

The amount of time spent in continuous aerobic movement should not exceed 15 minutes, according to ACOG. Use how you feel as a guideline for workout. A useful measure is Borg's Perceived Exertion Scale (see Table), since heart rate response itself may be variable and inconsistent.

The following chart is adapted from Swedish physiologist Gunnar Borg. Select a number within this range that best describes your level of exertion, and multiply that number by 10. The resulting product may be close to your working heart rate.

Scale of Perceived Exertion

20	Very, very hard
18	Very hard
16	Hard
14	Somewhat hard
12	Moderate
10	Light
8	Very light
6	Very, very light

Floor Work

The floor work portion of the class is important to the pregnant participant. A greater portion of the prenatal class is dedicated to floor work because (1) the exercises performed during floor work can directly relate to relaxation exercises for labor; (2) the time spent on gentle stretching and toning exercises can relieve much of the discomfort of pregnancy; and (3) floor work provides a stable base of support for exercise.

Abdominal exercises should not include any strain or feeling of "bearing down," which may occur in regular classes. The rectus abdominis muscle often has a normal midline separation during pregnancy. It's important to guard against further separation of this muscle by only doing modified abdominal work on hands and knees. Abdominal work should never be performed at a fast pace or with a sudden, jerky movement. A pelvic tilt, with the lower back pressed to the floor, should be maintained throughout abdominal curls.

A good alternative to abdominal curls is to get on all fours and gently pull the abdomen in and contract while exhaling. Make sure the back does not arch.

Inner and outer thigh work: Side leg lifts

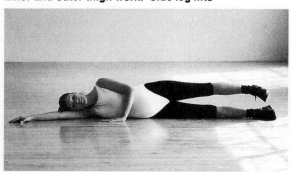 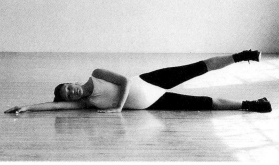

a.   b.

Abdominal curls with arm variation

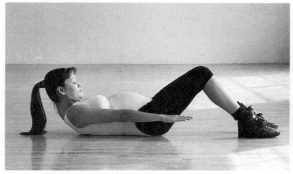

a. Arms at hips

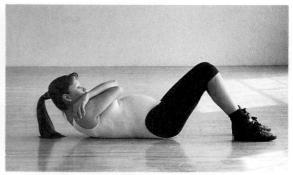

b. Arms crossed over chest

Alternative to abdominal curls

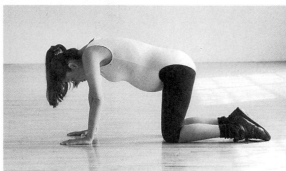

a. Contracting the abdomen

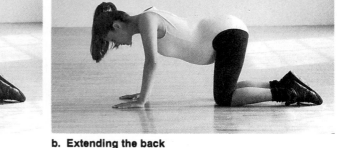

b. Extending the back

In advanced pregnancy, modify the abdominal work so that you roll back from an upright seated position to a backward lean of 45 degrees only. However, this movement primarily works the hip flexors, and the abdominals run a distant second.

Exercises for the back of the thigh should be reduced in number and intensity, if not eliminated. These exercises include extending and lifting the leg while in an all-fours position. The weight of the abdomen stresses the lower back when leg lifts are performed. Increased pressure on the diaphragm makes breathing difficult, and added strain is placed on the small, round ligaments near the groin.

Perform both inner and outer thigh work in the side-lying position, lying all the way down rather than up on your elbow. This keeps the spine in better alignment.

Cool-Down Stretches

Perform as many stretches on the floor as possible. In this way, you get the maximum support for your unstable posture. Instead of taking static stretches to the point of maximum resistance, do slow, controlled, relaxful stretching.

Floor work: Gentle limbering stretch

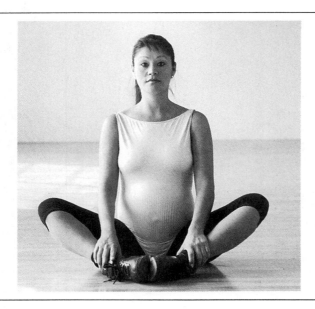

Make sure your heart rate is well below 60 percent of your maximum heart rate before getting on the floor for final floor work and cool-down stretches.

Special Exercises

Low-Impact Movement
Low-impact classes are definitely the way to go during pregnancy. Caution should be given to exaggerated upper body movement. Refrain from lifting the arms so high that the back arches and the abdomen protrudes even further.

Kegels
Muscles of the pelvic floor are not usually exercised in a regular aerobics class. Responsible for supporting the pelvic organs, these muscles hold the uterus floor in place and can prevent urinary incontinence and sexual dissatisfaction. The Kegel exercise, which strengthens these muscles located between the pubic bone in front and the coccyx in the back, should be emphasized in a pregnancy class. You can do this "invisible" little exercise by imagining the area at the base of your pubic region is like an elevator floor. When you contract the right muscles the elevator floor rises a few inches. These are the same muscles you use when you try to stop the flow of urine.

During pelvic tilts, incorporate the Kegel exercise to strengthen these muscles. Kegels should be done from early in the pregnancy through your lifetime.

Standing Work
It is recommended to warm up the lower back, midback, shoulders, and upper back before making any lateral, side-bending motions. A gentle head drop and forward shoulder roll can loosen tension in the upper body and back.

Standing waist work should be performed at half the speed of the regular repetitions. Never lean so far to the side that you lose your balance. Also, doing a stretch to one side with both arms overhead (double overhead arm side stretches) should never be done. Always lift upward with only a slight side bend when warming up the side muscles.

Upper body work for muscular endurance can be safely performed in a standing position as long as special attention is paid to proper body alignment. This means: knees should be soft, never locked; feet shoulder-width apart; toes pointing out slightly; hips tucked under slightly; rib cage lifted; abdominals held in to support the lower back; shoulders back and down; and head held high.

Controversial Exercises

Whether pregnant women should exercise on their backs is one of the most controversial issues in exercise and pregnancy. ACOG does not recommend exercises from a back position after the fourth month of pregnancy. Many physicians and other programs, including Pregnancy the Aerobic Way (PAW), disagree, reporting that many women sleep on their backs and labor on their backs without incident.

If you are pregnant and lying on your back, your blood vessels may be compressed, leading to a fall in blood pressure, dizziness, and fainting for you, and decreased oxygen for the fetus. If these symptoms arise, avoid back-lying exercises. If back-lying positions do not create a problem, PAW recommends that exercises under three minutes be performed. Roll to your side for a rest period before proceeding to the next exercise.

Exercises to Avoid

High Knee Lifts
High knee lifts create an irritation and soreness in the round ligaments that run diagonally down the sides of the pelvis and suspend the uterus in the pelvic cavity.

Quick Lateral Movements
Rapidly shifting direction with quick lateral movements can increase the chance of falling because your center of gravity is thrown off balance. Overly rapid lateral movements can also put a torque motion on the knees, causing strain and injury.

High-Impact Jumping and Jarring
High-impact movements are not recommended if you are pregnant. The increased weight adds to orthopedic injuries of the lower back, hips, knees, shins, ankles, and feet. Your altered center of gravity increases the risk of falling during jumping.

Turn a heel jack or jump kick into a step with heel out.

Weights
The use of wrist or ankle weights during pregnancy is not recommended. If pregnant, you are fully challenged by adjusting to the addition of 15 to 35

pounds. You need no further workload added to your already taxed musculoskeletal framework.

Traditional Rejects

Basically the same exercises that lead to injury in a regular aerobics class should be avoided if you are pregnant. These include plough, hurdler's stretch, full neck circles, standing toe touches, deep knee bends, double leg lifts, straight leg sit-ups, kneeling donkey kicks, deep leg lunges, and inverted bicycling. Most important, avoid all forward flexion unless your upper body weight is well supported.

Prone Position

Any prone (lying on the stomach) exercises are too uncomfortable and dangerous. Push-ups fall in this category.

Summary

1. In general, as long as a pregnant woman is in good health and has medical clearance from her physician, she can safely participate in a low-impact aerobic class.
2. Prenatal classes should be taught by trained professionals who are prepared to meet the physical and emotional needs of the pregnant exerciser.
3. Some important modifications can make the aerobics class a safe, enjoyable experience.
4. Warm-ups are often extended so that the changing orthopedic structure of the pregnant woman is adequately prepared. Both rhythmic limbering and mild walking are good warm-up exercises.
5. During cardiovascular work, the pregnant student is cautioned against a heart rate exceeding 140 beats per minute, or 80 percent of her maximum heart rate.
6. During floor work, part of the class may be devoted to relaxation exercises that help prepare for labor.
7. Alternatives to abdominal curls are important so that any normal separation of the rectus abdominis is not at risk in advanced stages of pregnancy.
8. Certain exercises such as Kegels, lower back stretches, and gentle groin stretches can alleviate much of the discomfort of pregnancy and add to the importance of a prenatal class.
9. Exercises that irritate and stress the supporting ligaments should be avoided.
10. Safety is the key factor for pregnant exercisers. An aerobics class not only should be safely modified, but should incorporate special exercises and adaptations to assure strength, endurance, flexibility, and well-being for both mother and fetus.

CHAPTER 10

Measuring Your Progress

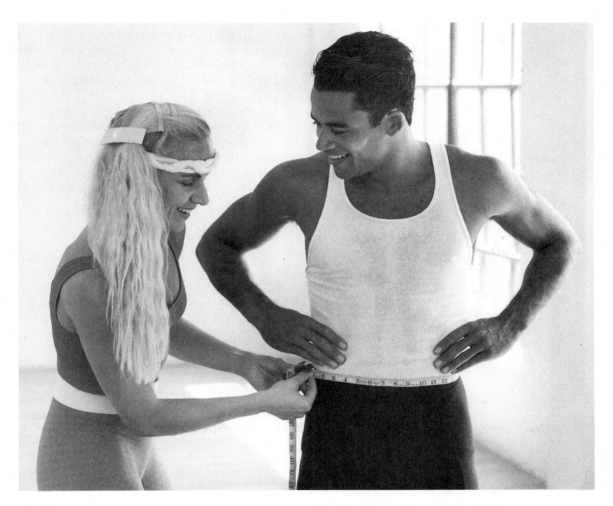

Outline

What Condition Are You In Now?
Assessing Your Personal Measurements
Testing Your Aerobic Capacity
   Modified Step Test
   Assessing Your Modified Step Test Score

Testing Your General Flexibility
Student Health History Form
Summary
Checklist: Semester Progress Chart

What Condition Are You In Now?

What condition are you in now? You may look pretty good in the mirror, but are you aerobically fit? Perhaps you are, but you're carrying a few extra pounds you would like to shed. It is important to evaluate your current fitness level so you: (1) are aware of your current status; and (2) can measure your progress. There is nothing better than seeing progress to help you stick with and enjoy a regular exercise program.

When you begin an exercise program, the initial discomforts of fatigue, soreness, dry mouth, and labored breathing seem discouraging. Try to remember there is no such thing as instant fitness. The benefits take about six to twelve weeks to appear. You must commit yourself to your exercise program. Unfortunately, if you are not committed and persistent, you may drop out before the results are apparent.

There is an easy way to visualize your progress. Gains, even small ones, can be measured right from the start. When you begin a new exercise program, take a good look at yourself in the mirror and assess your current fitness level so you can easily assess your progress. Becoming aware of your progress is a self-motivator and will help you stick to your exercise program. The three areas in which you can easily perform a self-assessment are personal measurements, flexibility, and aerobic conditioning.

Assessing Your Personal Measurements

It is sometimes difficult to take your own measurements because it can be awkward. Try to find a trusted friend to help you out and complete the following chart. If not, take your own measurements. Complete the chart before you begin your new aerobic exercise program, after 4 weeks into your exercise program, after 8 weeks, after 12 weeks, and after 16 weeks. You will be amazed at your progress!

Assessing Your Personal Measurements*

Area of Measurement	Beginning Date		4 weeks Date		8 weeks Date		12 weeks Date		16 weeks Date	
	Right	Left	Right	Left	Right	Left	Right	Left	Right	Left
Biceps/Triceps (upper arm midway between the elbow & shoulder joint)										
Chest										
Waist										
Hips (7" below the waist)										
Upper Thigh (feet approx. 12" apart; measure thighs 3" below crotch level)										
Calf										

*Note: Record your measurement to the closest 1/2 inch

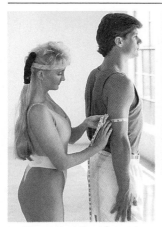

a. Measuring the biceps/
triceps area

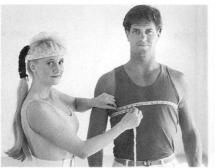

b. Measuring the chest

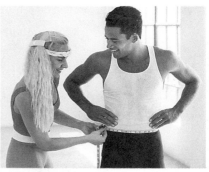

c. Measuring the waist

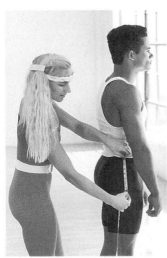

a. Locating 7" below waist
for hip measurement

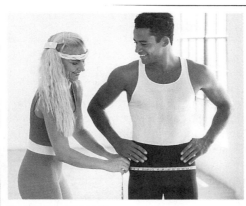

b. Hip measurment

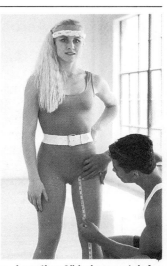

c. Locating 3" below crotch for
thigh measurement

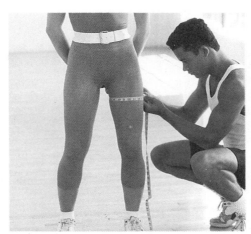

d. Upper thigh measurement

Measuring the calf

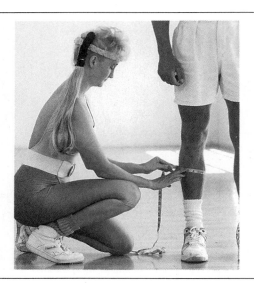

Testing Your Aerobic Capacity

Modified Step Test
You need a stopwatch, an 8-inch step (such as in the average staircase), and a chair to complete this test.

Directions: Step up and down, alternating feet, for 3 minutes at a rate of approximately 1 complete sequence every 2 seconds. Stop at exactly 3 minutes, and immediately sit in a chair. After 1 minute of rest, take your pulse for 30 seconds, and multiply it by 2 to obtain your 1-minute pulse recovery score.

Compare your 1-minute pulse recovery score to the following chart to find out your starting aerobic condition.

Training Heart Rates Chart

Heart Beats per Minute   Your score: _____

Age	Very High	High	Moderate	Low	Very Low
Female					
10–19	Below 82	82–91	92–97	98–102	Above 102
20–29	Below 83	83–87	88–93	94–98	Above 98
30–39	Below 83	82–89	90–95	96–98	Above 98
40–49	Below 83	82–87	88–97	98–102	Above 102
Over 50	Below 86	86–93	94–99	100–104	Above 104
Male					
10–19	Below 72	72–77	78–83	84–88	Above 89
20–29	Below 72	72–79	80–85	86–93	Above 94
30–39	Below 76	76–81	82–87	88–93	Above 94
40–49	Below 78	78–83	84–89	90–94	Above 95
Over 50	Below 80	80–85	86–91	92–95	Above 96

Modified step test

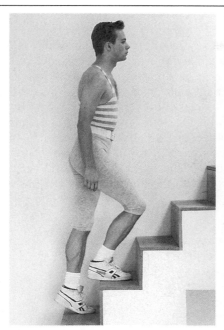

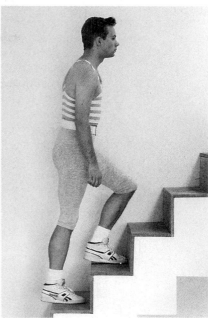

a.   b.

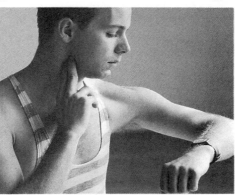

c. Taking pulse following step test

Assessing Your Modified Step Test Score

If you have been sedentary, your score will most likely be near 100 or slightly above, regardless of your age. If you are exceptionally fit, your score will be below that of someone your age who is less fit.

If your score on the modified step test is well below 100, and it falls within the very high or high rating, you already have a high cardiovascular respiratory endurance level. Keep up your good work!

If your score is within the moderate or low rating, there is room for improvement in your cardiovascular respiratory endurance level. If your score falls within the very low rating, a regular aerobic program will make a big difference in your cardiovascular respiratory endurance level.

Testing Your General Flexibility

Flexibility is specific to a joint or a combination of joints. With extensive testing, you can have the flexibility in every joint evaluated and identified. However, you can measure general flexibility by using the Sit and Reach Test. To perform this test, you need a Sit and Reach Box. Ask your instructor where you can find one or you can build one yourself (see appendix G).

Directions: Sit with the soles of your feet flat against the Sit and Reach Box. Keeping your knees straight, reach forward with your arms fully extended, palms down, fingers straight, and one hand on top of the other. Hold this position for 3 seconds. Repeat and use the best score.

Compare your score to the following chart to assess your flexibility.

Sit and Reach Flexibility Test						
Age	**17–19**	**20–29**	**30–39**	**40–49**	**50–59**	**60–65**
Males	centimeters					
Excellent	>48	>45	>45	>43	>42	>41
Good	37–48	37–44	34–44	32–42	31–41	29–40
Minimum	26–36	25–35	25–33	22–31	19–30	18–28
Below Min.	15–25	15–24	14–23	11–21	8—18	6–17
Poor	<14	<14	<12	<10	<7	<5
Females	centimeters					
Excellent	>43	>41	>38	>35	>32	>28
Good	39–42	38–40	35–37	32–34	28–31	25–27
Minimum	37–39	34–37	31–34	28–30	23–26	21–24
Below Min.	34–36	31–33	28–30	24–27	19–22	18–20
Poor	<33	<30	<27	<23	<17	<16

*Note: Footline set at 25 centimeters

Sit and reach test

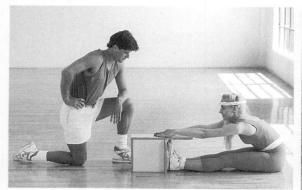

a.

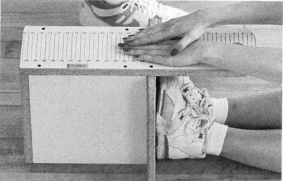

b. **Reading score of sit and reach test**

Student Health History

Before you begin your aerobics program, it is important for your instructor to know something about your history to assist you if necessary. Please fill out the form below, and give it to your instructor by the second week of class.

Name_____ Age_____
Date_____ Class Section_____

1. Do you have any of the following illnesses/conditions?

   _____ Asthma   _____ Epilepsy   _____ Hypertension
   _____ Emphysema   _____ Diabetes   _____ Heart Disease
   _____ Chest pain or discomfort   _____ Are you pregnant?

2. Have you had any of the following within the past 2 years?

   _____ Heart attack   _____ Stroke
   _____ Heart surgery   _____ Back injury
   _____ General major surgery. If so, please specify _____

3. Do you smoke? _____ Yes   _____ No

4. Are you currently taking any medications? _____ Yes _____ No
   If yes, please specify. _____

5. Are you currently under a doctor's care?   _____ Yes _____ No
   If yes, please specify the reason._____

6. Date of your last physical examination._____

7. According to your physician and/or charts, are you
   _____ Overweight   If so, by how much?_____
   _____ Underweight   If so, by how much?_____
   _____ Normal?

8. Do you have any handicaps or current or chronic injuries that limit your physical abilities? _____ Yes _____ No
   If so, please describe. _____

9. Please supply any additional information that might be helpful to your instructor. _____

10. What are your main goals of this class? (Rank them by placing a 1, 2, or 3 on the line next to your goal.)
    _____Lose weight   _____ Stay the same   _____Gain weight
    _____Tone muscles   _____ Build muscles   _____Lose inches
    _____Increase cardiovascular fitness
    _____Other (please describe)_____

    _____
    _____

Summary

1. You must assess your current fitness level so you can set goals for yourself and measure your progress.
2. Remember, there is no such thing as instant fitness. It takes six to twelve weeks of consistent participation in an aerobics class before you will see results.
3. Regularly fill out the chart entitled Assessing Your Personal Measurements so you can visualize your results.
4. Complete the Modified Step Test several times throughout the semester to evaluate your aerobic fitness level. Watch your improvement!
5. Be sure to perform the Sit and Reach Test to see your progress.
6. Fill out the Semester Progress Chart at the appropriate time to get an overall view of your progress.
7. Now you are on the road to improving your fitness and feeling better. Congratulations!

 Checklist: Semester Progress Chart

It is valuable to identify your progress throughout the semester. Complete the following for each week listed.

Progress Chart

	Week 1		Week 8		Week 10		Week 15	
Weight								
Waist Measurement								
	R	L	R	L	R	L	R	L
Upper Arm Measurement (Around bicep/tricep muscle area)								
Thigh Measurement (3" below crotch)								
Hip Measurement (7" below waist)								
Resting Heart Rate								
Sit and Reach Flexibility								
Modified Step Test								
Maximum Number of Push-ups								
Number of Curl-ups in 1 Minute								

CHAPTER 11

Selecting a Class

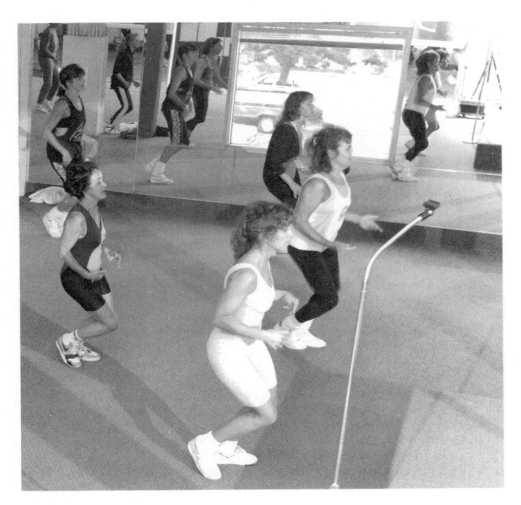

Outline

What to Look for in a Good Instructor
Characteristics of a Good Instructor
The Aerobic Dance Exercise Class
Selecting a Facility
Checklist for Selecting a Facility
Summary

What to Look for in a Good Instructor

When you think about signing up for a dance exercise class, you wonder where to begin. There are many teachers to choose from and many places to take classes. Some people erroneously think that if the instructor looks good, then that person must be a good instructor. Unfortunately, many establishments employ instructors based on their appearance instead of their qualifications. After reading this chapter, you will know the right questions to ask to seek out a qualified instructor. If you take classes from a qualified instructor, you will be able to get the most out of your workout.

Characteristics of a Good Instructor

Good instructors teach with enthusiasm and genuine concern for their students. They come to class well prepared to teach and arrive in ample time to set up the room and begin on time. An instructor should always start a class promptly and finish on time. Before the series of classes begins, a good instructor explains the goals of aerobics, how and why to take your pulse, and how to determine your target heart range. A good aerobics instructor should be a role model, a person who is fit and who lives a healthy lifestyle. This does not mean that your instructor should look like he or she walked off the cover of a magazine—not all good instructors look like movie stars. Other very important characteristics of a good instructor are that he or she has a professional affiliation with an educational resource organization and demonstrates a commitment to continuing education. Your instructor should have a fitness certificate or an equivalent certification from a university or a private certifying organization.

It is very important for your safety that your instructor shows a knowledge of appropriate applications of exercise physiology and injury prevention by demonstrating only safe and effective exercise techniques. Also, your instructor should be able to modify the exercises for those with special needs, such as the overweight or pregnant exerciser. Another very important certification that your instructor should have is cardiopulmonary resuscitation (CPR).

Does the instructor conduct the class in a nonintimidating and noncompetitive manner? That's how a good class should be conducted. Is he or she there for a personal workout or for YOU? Is the instructor conscious of how the environment is affecting the class? Is it too hot or too cold? Is the music too loud? Are people bumping into one another? A good instructor will be cognizant of these factors and make the appropriate adjustments. The instructor should be aware of the fatigue level of the class and look for signs of overexertion. Similarly, individuals who appear not to be working hard enough might need encouragement.

The Aerobic Dance Exercise Class

Every instructor has a unique style—and that's good! However, all classes should follow basically the same formula. First, there should be a 7- to 10-minute warm-up that includes all major muscle groups and avoids ballistic stretches. Following the warm-up is the aerobics section of class, which lasts

15 to 30 minutes depending on the length of the class. During this time, there should be a gradual build-up, a sustained high-intensity level, and a gradual decrease in intensity. Finally, it is important to have the post-aerobics cool-down where intensity gradually decreases so as not to shock the system with a sudden change of pace. Your instructor should guide you in checking your pulse rate 5 minutes into the aerobics and at the end of the aerobics section. There should also be a post-aerobic recovery check 2 to 3 minutes after cool-down.

The organization of the dance exercises should flow smoothly and skillfully from one movement to another and one section of class to the other. The cues given by the instructor should be easily understood, and the movements should be challenging and keep your interest. Too much time spent on one activity without variation leads to boredom. A good instructor changes the movements frequently yet allows enough repetition so you can eventually be successful.

A good class also includes about 15 minutes of exercises to strengthen the muscles of the arms, chest, shoulders, abdomen, back, legs, buttocks, and hips. A 5-minute cool-down includes static stretches for every muscle group worked.

Selecting a Facility

A good facility or club makes you feel good about yourself and makes you want to return to work out again. A well-run facility is concerned about your welfare and not only your membership. A qualified, concerned director hires only qualified instructors and makes sure they are familiar with the equipment and safety skills. A good facility maintains a clean, hygienic environment. The showers, restrooms, and locker rooms are clean and well maintained. The temperature is well regulated in the workout and dressing area. A good facility has a suspended or coiled wood floor, high-density matting, or absorbent flooring material in the aerobics room.

If the facility has weight equipment, the area should be effectively supervised with qualified leaders. The equipment should be well maintained and in good working order. Policies should be established and enforced to allow all members easy accessibility to the equipment. A facility with weight training equipment should be set up so you can keep a log of your progress and file it in the workout area for easy accessibility each time you exercise.

When selecting the facility, be sure to check the schedule of classes. Does it offer classes at times you can attend? If it doesn't, the facility won't be of much use to you. Does it demonstrate a willingness to adapt to the clients' requests for different time slots, more classes, and a variety of offerings for example, low-impact, prenatal, and high-impact? Are other services available, such as a nutritionist, physical therapy, massage, and a referral network of physicians in case of injury? Is the facility convenient to your home or work? Does it provide child care facilities? Does the membership fee fit into your budget?

All of these considerations should be well evaluated when selecting a facility. Select the facility that best meets your needs. If you don't, you may find you have joined a club you won't really use. So take time to investigate the facility before you join. It will save you money and aggravation in the future.

Checklist for Selecting a Facility

1. Is it conveniently located?
2. Are there classes given at the times you desire?
3. What is the composition of the aerobics floor? Is it shock absorbent?
4. Are there weight-training facilities?
5. What are the qualifications of the instructors for aerobics and for weight training?
6. Are there other facilities, such as weights or a swimming pool?
7. What social activities are offered (socials, dances, trips, tournaments)?
8. Can you afford the membership fee?

Summary

1. Your most important consideration is the instructor you choose for your class.
2. A good instructor:
   - Is certified by an accredited organization and/or is university trained.
   - Holds a CPR (cardiopulmonary resuscitation) card.
   - Arrives on time and begins on time.
   - Is clear and thorough about the goals of the class.
   - Assists you in finding your target heart rate.
   - Conducts the class in a nonintimidating manner.
3. Characteristics of an effective class:
   - 7 to 10 minutes of warm-up.
   - 15 to 30 minutes of aerobic work that keeps you at your target heart rate.
   - 3 to 5 minute aerobic cool-down
   - Approximately 15 minutes of strength development and toning.
   - 5 minutes of cool-down activities and flexibility.
4. A facility should have:
   - A soft floor (suspended or coiled-wood floor), absorbent flooring, or mats.
   - Clean and well-maintained areas.
   - Classes at convenient times.

CHAPTER 12

A Guide to Buying Media for Personal Use

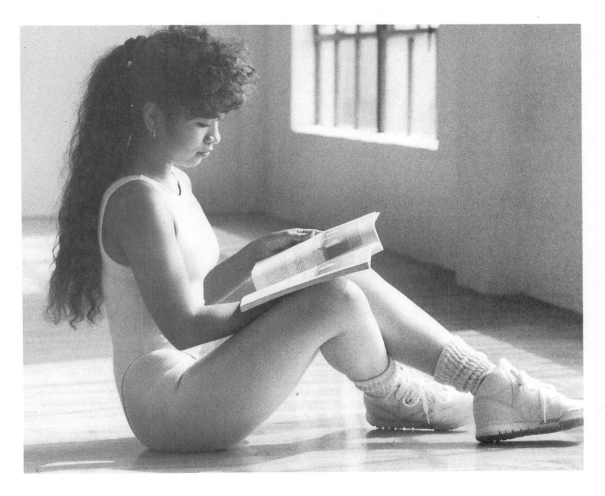

Outline

Selecting a Videotape
Evaluating a Videotape
Purchasing a Videotape
Checklist: Videotape Evaluation
Selecting Music to Create Your Own Routines
Summary

You may find that occasionally you have to miss an exercise class and you'll need to work out at home or in a motel room while you are traveling. To prepare for that situation you could buy a videotape (for home use) or music (to use at home or when traveling) to motivate you through your own routine. Here are some guidelines for buying your media.

Selecting a Videotape

There are over 150 aerobics videotapes on the market from which to choose. The videotapes vary in ability level and style. However, for the most part, these home video workouts attempt to offer you a safe, effective, informative exercise program that you can execute at any location. Some videos simply present the exercise material, others give you extensive scenery and elaborate camera angles. Before you purchase a videotape, preview it or rent it so you can evaluate whether it meets your needs.

Evaluating a Videotape

In evaluating a videotape for purchase, rate the following five areas as they relate to your needs: instructor technique, balance and flow of the class, safety, technical proficiency of the production, and the overall effectiveness of the videotape for your purposes.

Checklist: Videotape Evaluation

After viewing the videotape, check the *yes* or *no* column for each question. Once you have completed the checklist, add up your *yes* responses and your *no* responses. If you have significantly more *yes* responses, the videotape is acceptable.

Instructor Technique   Yes No

1. Does the instructor give adequate cues to guide you into the movement? ☐ ☐
2. Can you follow the choreography? ☐ ☐
3. Do you like the choreography? ☐ ☐
4. Are the transitions smooth? ☐ ☐

Class Balance   Yes No

1. Does the class include all five parts of a good lesson: warm-up, aerobics, aerobic cool-down, strength and flexibility, and an overall cool-down? ☐ ☐

2. Is the time allotted to each section of the class properly balanced?　☐　☐
   Warm-up: 7 to 10 minutes
   Aerobics: 15 to 30 minutes
   Aerobic Cool-down: 5 minutes
   Strengthening and Toning: 15 minutes
   Overall Cool-down and Flexibility: 5 minutes
3. Is the entire body worked out in the routine?　☐　☐

Safety Information

1. Does the instructor discuss proper body alignment and or proper ways to execute each exercise?　☐　☐
2. Are the demonstrations executed with proper body alignment?　☐　☐
3. Is there an accompanying guide book that discusses exercise precautions?　☐　☐
4. Is time alloted to check your target heart rate?　☐　☐

Technical Proficiency

1. Are the camera angles appropriate for you to understand the movement?　☐　☐
2. Do the camera angles assist your learning or detract from it?　☐　☐
3. Is is difficult to follow the movement because of the way it is photographed?　☐　☐
4. Is the music well recorded?　☐　☐
5. Do you like the music?　☐　☐
6. Is the cuing properly coordinated with the demonstration?　☐　☐

Overall Effectiveness

1. Does the videotape provide you with a model you can follow?　☐　☐
2. Is the videotape presentation of the class motivating to you?　☐　☐
3. Did you enjoy exercising to the tape?
4. Did the tape provide you with the workout you need?　☐　☐
   Total number of YES responses_____
   Total number of NO responses_____

   Did you have more *yes* responses than *no* responses?　☐　☐
   After evaluating a videotape, review the checklist. If the responses are mostly positive, the tape should work for you. If the responses are mostly negative, keep reviewing videotapes until you find one that meets your needs.

Purchasing a Videotape

With such a wide selection available, it is highly probable that your local vendor doesn't carry all of them. First, investigate what tapes your local vendor carries, find out whether you can preview them or at least rent them. Check out the supply at another vendor and again see whether you can preview the tapes of your choice. Use the Checklist for Evaluation on the previous page to help you make your selection. Since you will be using the tape more than once, it is important that it meets your needs and that you are satisfied with it before you purchase it. A catalog is available that describes most of the exercise tapes on the market. It may be worth sending for it before you purchase a videotape. To order your free catalog, send your name and address to:

Video Exercise Catalog
Department M
5390 Main Street NE
Minneapolis, MN 55421

Selecting Music to Create Your Own Routines

When creating your own routines, you need to decide what music to use. The simplest solution, of course, is to use music you already have. However, the tempo won't necessarily be appropriate for the exercises you want to do. You can spend hours attempting to find the right music.

Several companies sell music for aerobics—they have adjusted the tempo of contemporary songs to fit warm-up, aerobics, strength and flexibility exercises, and cool-down. Here are several of the companies from which you can order music for aerobics:

Dance Tracks
72 Spring Street
Suite 1004
New York, NY 10012

Music In Motion
P. O. Box 2688
Alameda, CA 94501

East Coast Music Productions, Inc.
P. O. Box 3812
Gaithersburg, MD 20878

Summary

1. Sometimes it is difficult for you to attend a dance exercise class, so you may like to have an aerobics videotape to follow on your own time.
2. Before you purchase a videotape, evaluate it for quality and suitability.
3. There are more than 150 videotapes on the market for exercising at home or when you are traveling.
4. You may want to purchase taped music to perform *your* personal workout when you are travelling or when you can't get to class.

CHAPTER 13

Being Creative: Choreographing Your Own Routines

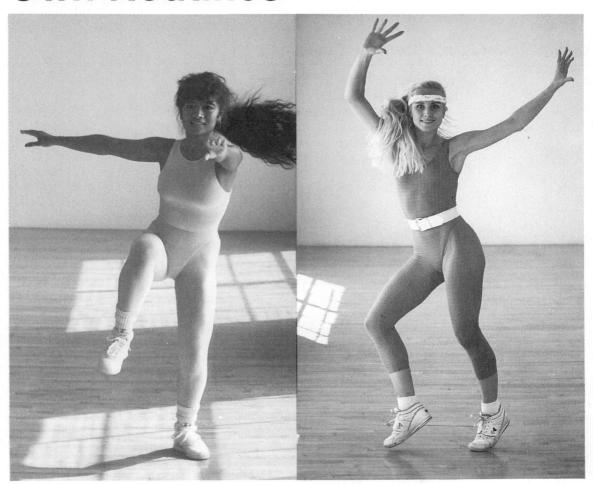

Outline

Creating Your Dance Exercise Routine
Checklist: Creating a Routine
Simple 8-Count Phrases of Movement
Summary

Many students like to create (choreograph) their own dance exercise routines to music they enjoy. Choreographing your own routines can be a very creative and satisfying experience. Before you begin, remember that the goal of aerobic dance exercise is to combine dance steps and movement patterns, coordinated with music, that keep you moving continuously so you can exercise your body and heart. The workout should be 15 to 30 minutes long, allowing you to reach your target heart rate and receive the exercise training effect you desire. If you want high-impact routines, use movements that have a lot of bounce. If you want low-impact routines, keep one foot in contact with the floor at all times.

Creating Your Dance Exercise Routine

First, select your music. The music should have a steady beat as well as a motivating "up beat" feeling that makes you want to work hard. Once you select your music, listen to it and analyze the musical phrasing. Usually, the music is composed such that you can create phrases of movement that take 8 counts. You can create several phrases of 8 counts of movement and then combine them in various ways to "fit" the composition of the music. Each phrase you create can be given a letter to identify it. If you create 4 phrases, letter them A, B, C, and D. Then combine the phrases in any order you like; for example, A B C D A B A B C D. The phrases can be repeated in any order, and as many times as you desire, as long as they fit with the music.

You don't have to be a dancer to create an enjoyable, high-energy routine. An example of 4 phrases of movement (identified as A, B, C, and D) that you could combine into a routine is:

A: Hop on the left foot 4 times while pointing and tapping the right foot forward and then to the side (for example, forward, side, forward, feet together on count 4, jump/change sides). Repeat the entire phrase while hopping (bouncing) on the right foot 4 times and tapping the left foot forward and to the side as described. Repeat the phrase again on each side.

Phrase A: Hop on left foot (a) while pointing and tapping right foot (b) foward and to the side

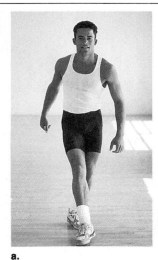 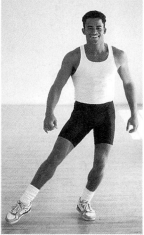

a.   b.

Phrase B: Run and clap

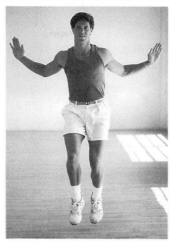
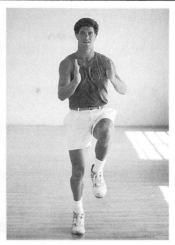

a.   **b.**

B: Run in place 8 times, clap on each run.
C: Do 8 jumping jacks using full arm movements.
D: Slide to the right 8 times, clap on the 8th slide. Repeat to the left.

    These phrases can be first performed in the A B C D format and then combined in any order you feel works well with the movement. A simple way to add variety is to do different arm movements each time you repeat the phrase. When you make a variation, identify that lettered phrase with a subscript number. For example, let's say the original phrase is lettered "A." The next time you repeat "A" but vary the arm movements, identify the phrase as "A_1." Your new routine might be: A B C D A_1 B_1 C_1 D_1 A B C D.

    In this routine, you use the original 4 phrases, change the arm movements that accompany each phrase, then repeat the original 4 phrases of movement. A more challenging and diversified routine has more than 4 phrases to combine.

Phrase D: Slide and clap on last one

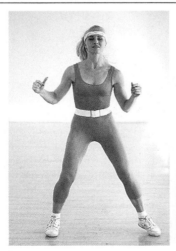
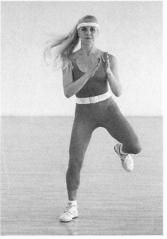

a.   **b.**

Checklist: Creating a Routine

1. You will be creating a dance exercise routine that lasts 15 to 30 minutes and is of high enough intensity to keep your heart rate in the training zone during your entire routine.
2. Select music.
3. Create an 8-count phrase of movement. This is your "A" phrase.
4. Create another 8-count phrase of movement. This is your "B" phrase.
5. Create your "C" phrase of movement. Again, this consists of 8 counts.
6. Create your 8-count phrase of movement to be called "D."
7. Practice the movement in phrases A, B, C, and D, letting each phrase follow the previous one.
8. Try to do your A B C D movements with the music. At this point, you may need to modify your movements to make them flow with the music.
9. Decide how you would like to complete your routine. Do you want to repeat the A B C D phrase in order, or do you want to vary the order? After you have decided, perform the A B C D phrase, and follow it with your next set of movements (for example, C D A B).
10. Practice doing your routine with the music.
11. Create another routine by following the steps just listed. Continue this process until you have created enough routines to give yourself a 15- to 30-minute workout.
12. Have fun, and HAPPY WORKOUT!

It is up to you how many phrases you would like to create and use in each routine. Movement phrases longer than 8 counts may be difficult for you to remember at the beginning. However, when you become more experienced you can challenge yourself and create longer routines and utilize more complex movements.

The phrases you use in your dance exercise routines are only limited by your abilities and creativity. So, have fun and create the routines to which you would like to exercise!

You can use the following 8-count phrases of movement in any order in creating your own dance exercise routines. These are only representative of the types of steps you can use; there is really no limit to the phrases you can create. Be creative and have fun!

Simple 8-Count Phrases of Movement

- Jump in place 8 times while hitting the sides of your thighs with straight arms.
- Walk in place on your toes, performing 16 steps while moving your arms down and up on the sides or in front of your body.

Jump in place while hitting thighs

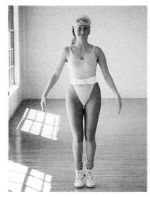 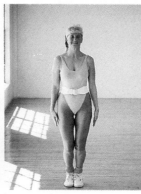

a.   b.

Walking in place

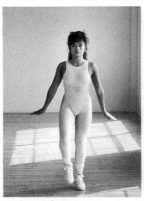 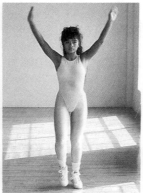

a. Arms down   b. Arms up

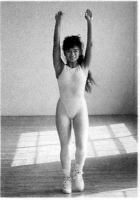 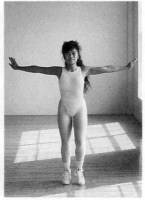

c. Arms up and front   d. Arms halfway down

Running in place while lifting feet high

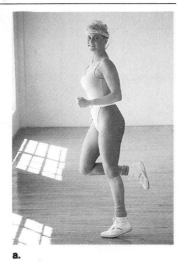

a.

Running in place while lifting knees high

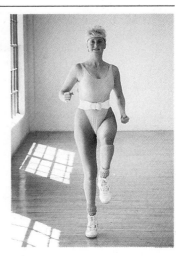

- Run in place 8 times while lifting your feet high in the rear.
- Run in place 8 times while lifting your knees high in front.
- Perform 8 jumping jacks, moving your arms down and up in coordination with the leg movements.
- Perform 8 jumping jacks, moving your arms down and only half way up (to the shoulder level) in coordination with each leg movement.

Jumping jacks

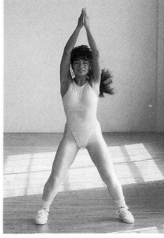

a.

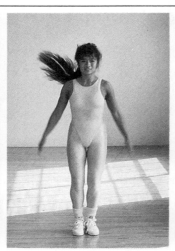

b.

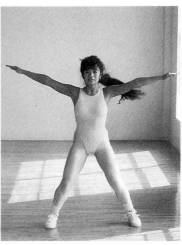

c.

Mountain climber

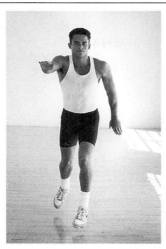 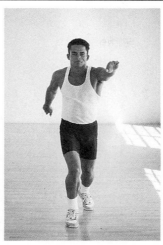 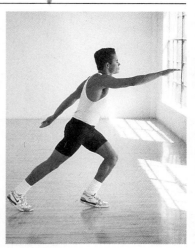

a.   b.   c. **Side view**

- Mountain Climber: With your feet separated, jump and land forward and backward a distance of about one foot. Alternate feet as you land in front and in back on each jump. Your arms can swing high in opposition to the leg movements.
- Pony: "Hop, step, step." Hop on the right foot to the side, then quickly step with the left foot and then the right foot. Repeat on the other side.

Pony

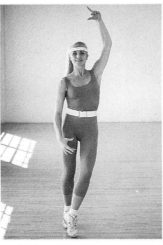 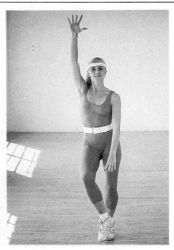

a.   b.

Heel, toe, slide, slide

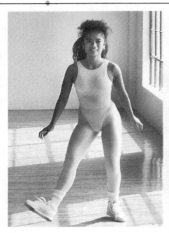 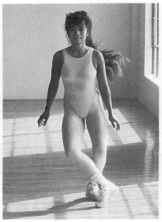 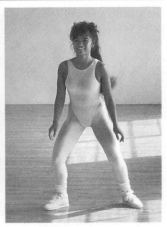

a.   b.   c.

- Heel, toe, slide, slide: Hop on the left foot while tapping the right heel to the right side. While hopping again on the left foot, swing the right foot to the front and touch the toe on the floor. Perform 2 slides to the right. Repeat the entire phrase by hopping on the right foot and sliding to the left.
- Hop on one foot and lift up the opposite knee. Reverse.
- Hop on one foot, and swing kick the opposite foot forward. Reverse.
- Charleston Bounce Step: Use a very bouncy step throughout this phrase. Step right, kick the left foot forward, step back on the left foot, and touch the right toe back. Repeat 8 times. Reverse.
- Can-Can Kick: Hop on the right foot, and simultaneously bring the bent left knee up high in front. Hop again on the right foot, lightly touch the left foot on the floor next to the right, and kick the left foot into the air. Repeat 4 times and then repeat on the other side. A more advanced version involves alternating sides after each kick.

Hop on one foot, swing kick opposite foot

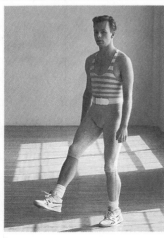 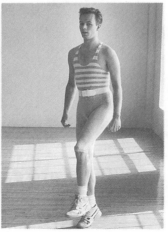

a.   b.

Hop on one foot and swing kick the other side

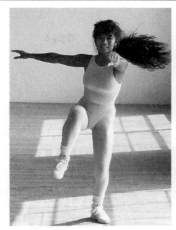
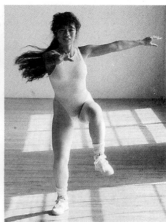

a.   b.

Charleston bounce step

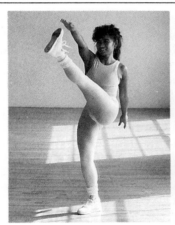
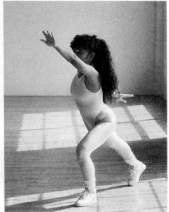

a.   b.

Can-can kick

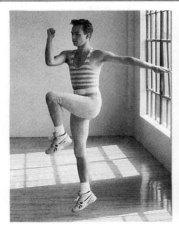
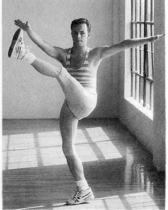

a.   b.

Schottische

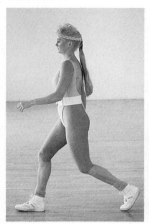
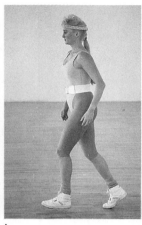
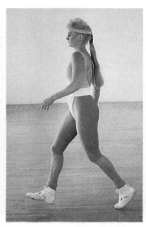
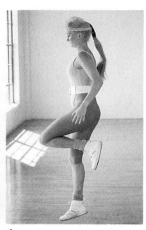

a.   b.   c.   d.

- Schottische: Run 3 times in place or while traveling, and hop and clap simultaneously (Run R, L, R, hop R). Alternate sides 4 times.
- Grapevine: While traveling to the right, cross left foot over the right, step to the right on the right foot, cross the left foot behind the right, and step on the right foot while traveling to the right. Repeat this phrase 4 times, moving to the right. To perform the grapevine in reverse with a smooth transition, begin by stepping on the left foot to the left before crossing the right foot over the left.

Grapevine

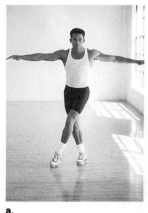
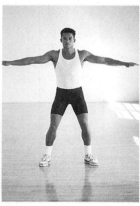
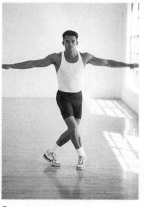
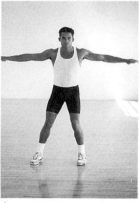

a.   b.   c.   d.

Grapevine schottische

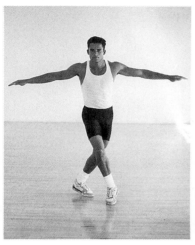 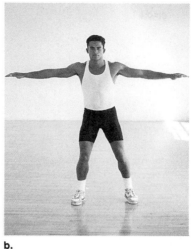 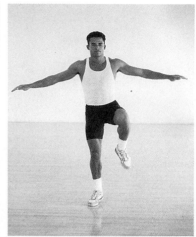

a.   b.   c.

- Grapevine schottische: Step to the right on the right foot, cross the left foot behind the right, step on the right to the right, and hop on the right. To reverse, step on the left foot to the left, cross the right foot behind the left, step on the left foot to the left, and hop on the left foot. Repeat 4 times.
- Run 3 times in place, and kick and clap on the 4th count. Alternate sides. Repeat the phrase 4 times.

Run 3 times in place, and kick and clap on the 4th count

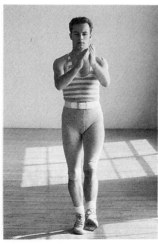 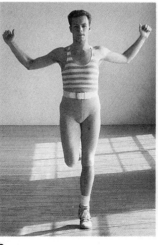 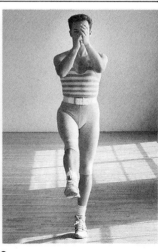

a.   b.   c.

Twisting the body

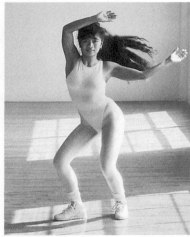 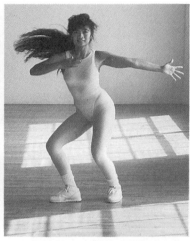 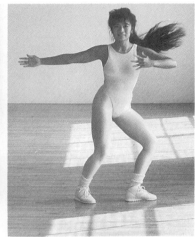

a. **Arms overhead**   b. **Arms side to side at chest level**   c.

- Twist the body while using a bounce landing, and swing the arms in opposition overhead on each twist. The arms can also be swung from side to side at chest level.
- Jump kick: Jump and kick the right foot forward, jump and kick the left foot forward. Vary the movement by kicking the leg on a diagonal and alternating the direction of the kick. Perform 8 jump kicks, alternating sides.

Jump kick

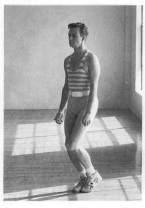 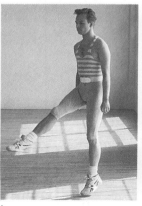 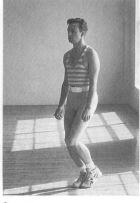 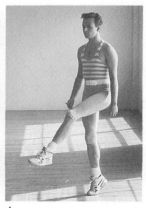

a.   b.   c.   d.

Skiers' jump

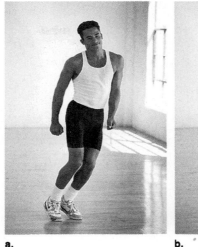 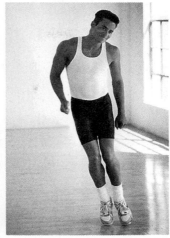

a.   b.

- Skiers' jump: Jump to the right while twisting the body toward the left diagonal. Reverse on the other side. Perform 8 times. For variety, you can jump twice on each side before changing directions.

Summary

1. Many students like to choreograph their own routines. They find it a creative experience to create routines to music they enjoy.
2. The aerobic routine you create should last 15 to 30 minutes and be strenuous enough to allow you to reach your target heart rate.
3. Select music that motivates you and has a steady beat.
4. Create movement phrases consisting of 8 counts each. Label each phrase with a letter, such as A B C and D. Then combine the lettered phrases the way they best fit the music, for example, A B C D A C D D B A. There is no limit to the way you can combine your movements. Have fun!
5. Remember to monitor your heart rate every five minutes to see whether you are staying in your target heart rate zone.

CHAPTER 14

Becoming an Instructor

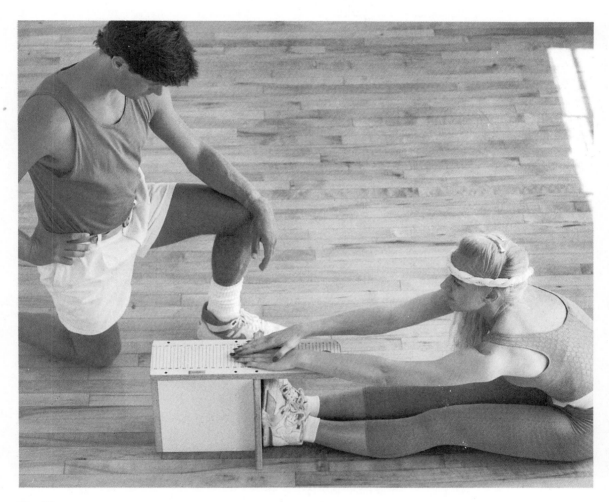

Outline

Where to Study to Become an Instructor
Checklist: Do I Want to Be an Instructor?
Summary

Many people who have taken aerobic dance classes for a long time wonder what it takes to become a dance exercise instructor. To become an instructor, you must first enjoy aerobics. Second, you must be in top physical condition. Third, you must study exercise physiology, anatomy and kinesiology, nutrition and weight control, components of teaching aerobic dance exercise, and first aid and cardiopulmonary resuscitation. Finally, you must enjoy working with and helping people.

There is a movement in this country to require all aerobic dance exercise instructors to be certified. However, at this point, there is no such national mandate. The certification requirement rests with each state or private agency. At present, no state requires dance exercise instructors to be state-certified or nationally certified. Many universities offer fitness instructor certificates that are recognized by hiring agencies. Many firms require their instructors to be certified, which is a sign of a responsible organization.

Consumers deserve to be taught by the very best person available. If a class is taught by someone who is good looking but uneducated, the participants risk being injured and the organization risks a law suit. Many dance exercise participants are well educated, and they may stop attending a class taught by an uneducated instructor. It is to an agency's advantage to hire well-trained instructors. Thus, if you would like to become an instructor, start taking classes and studying.

Where to Study to Become an Instructor

Many universities and colleges offer fitness instructor certificates in courses taught by well-educated, knowledgeable instructors. If your local university does not offer a certificate program, your next source is a private agency. There are over fifty private organizations offering fitness instructor certificates or dance exercise instructor certificates. The quantity and quality of instruction vary greatly from one organization to the next. You must thoroughly investigate the courses and the time you will spend in each. Make sure there are course offerings in the following subjects:

- Exercise Physiology
- Anatomy and Kinesiology
- Nutrition and Weight Control
- Components of Teaching Aerobic Dance Exercise
- Health Screening, and Modifying for Individual Variations
- First Aid
- Cardiopulmonary Resuscitation

Since there are so many private organizations and colleges offering certificates, it is hard to choose one. The decision is yours; you must study the options available to you.

The four largest and most recognized private agency certifications are offered through:

The Aerobics and Fitness Association of America
15250 Ventura Boulevard, Suite 310
Sherman Oaks, CA 91403
(818) 905-0040

Checklist: Do I Want to Be an Instructor?

1. Am I interested in leading and helping other people?
2. Am I good at motivating people?
3. Am I liked by many people?
4. Can I express myself well?
5. Do I have the desire, time, and money to go to school to study to become an instructor?
6. Am I willing to study for the courses necessary to become an instructor?

   If you answered "yes" to these questions, maybe you would make a good instructor. Perhaps it is time for you to investigate the local schools and/or organizations that certify dance exercise instructors.

American College of Sports Medicine
P. O. Box 1440
Indianapolis, IN 40206
(317) 637-9200

International Dance Exercise Association Foundation
6190 Cornerstone Court East, Suite 202
San Diego, CA 92121
(619) 535-8227

Y.M.C.A.
101 N. Walker Drive
Chicago, IL 60606
(312) 269-0516

If you do decide to become an aerobic dance instructor, it is imperative that you take course, in the subjects mentioned. You want to do the best job you can as an instructor. To do that, you must be well qualified and educated in all aspects of teaching aerobic dance exercise. Good luck to you!

Summary

1. To become an aerobic dance instructor, you must enjoy this kind of exercise and enjoy motivating people.
2. You need to be in top physical condition to be an aerobics instructor.
3. You must study many subjects so you will be well prepared to be the best instructor you possibly can. The subjects you will need to study are physiology, anatomy and kinesiology, nutrition and weight control, components of teaching aerobic dance exercise, and first aid and cardiopulmonary resuscitation.
4. Investigate the various places you can study to become an instructor. Both universities and private agencies offer programs.
5. Good luck to you, and happy studying!

Apparel

Alitta
75 Spring St., New York, NY 10012
(212) 334-1390

Apparel Warehouse
18318 Oxnard St., Tarzana, CA 91356
(818) 344-3224

Ballet Makers, Inc.
One Campus Rd., Totowa, NJ 07512
(201) 595-9000

Body Basics
910 E. Walnut, Washington, IL 61571
(309) 444-7538

Body Wrappers
25 W. 31st St., New York, NY 10001
(212) 570-1088

Cabriole
57 Smith Pl., Cambridge, MA 02138
(617) 492-3931

Carushka
15414 Cabrito Rd., #B, Van Nuys, CA 91406
(818) 904-0574

Dance France
2503 Main St., Santa Monica, CA 90405
(213) 392-9786

Danskin
111 W. 40th St., 18th Floor, New York, NY 10018
(212) 930-9121

Designer Sport
10000 Canoga Ave., Suite C-6,
Chatsworth, CA 91311
(818) 700-1040

Eurotard
1328 Union Hill Rd., Alpharetta, GA 30201
(404) 998-5675

Finelines Exercise Wear
294 Wilson Ave., Toronto, Ontario M3H 1S8
(416) 631-6828

Gilbert Apparel Group
P. O. Box 990, Edwards, CO 81632
(303) 926-2124

Graphic Jackets
727 NW Westover Terrace, Portland, OR 97210
(503) 295-1987

Heavenly Bodies
35070 E. 2nd Ave., Vancouver, VST 1B1,
Canada

High Country Fashions
8120 Penn Ave. S., #446,
Bloomington, MN 55431

Hind
390 Buckley Rd., San Luis Obispo, CA 93401
(805) 544-8555

International Male
2800 Midway Dr., San Diego, CA 92110

Jog-Bra Inc.
One Mill St., Burlington, VT 05401
(802) 863-3548

Kicks Bodywear
200 Sardis Road No., Matthews, NC 28105
(704) 847-7570

Marika
301 Spruce St., San Diego, CA 92103
(619) 295-4124

Gilda Marx Industries
11755 Exposition Blvd., Los Angeles, CA 90064
(213) 473-0872

Mazeppa
11044 Weddington St.
North Hollywood, CA 91601
(213) 273-5778

Jacques Moret
1350 Broadway, New York, NY 10018
(212) 736-0041

New Motion
2699 E. 28th St., #412, Signal Hill, CA 90806
(213) 427-5404

Oakbrook Hosiery
1750 Merrick Ave., Merrick, NY 11566
(516) 546-5800

Physical Fashions
289 Allwood Rd., Clifton, NJ 07012
(201) 376-1060

Rainbeau
150 7th St., San Francisco, CA 94103
(415) 431-0205

Schatzi
1283 Boulevard Way, Walnut Creek, CA 94595
(415) 943-1199

H.W. Shaw, Inc.
P. O. Box 4034, Hollywood, FL 33083
(800) 327-9548

Softouch
1167 N.W. 159th Dr., Miami, FL 33169
(305) 624-5581

The Sport Club
615 W. Johnson Ave., Cheshire, CT 06410
(800) 345-3610

Taffy's
701 Beta Dr., Cleveland, OH 44143
(216) 461-3360

Wags Motionwear
106 Dunster Rd., Jamaica Plain, MA 02130
(800) 543-3013

Workout Designs
14841 Velie Way, Suite F, Palm Desert, CA 92261
(800) 445-4379

Associations and Organizations

Academy for Myotherapy and Physical Fitness
9 School St., Lenox, PA 01240
(413) 637-0317

Aerobic Way
403 Navajo, Lake Quivira, KS 66106
(913) 268-9812

Aerobics and Fitness Association of America
15250 Ventura Blvd., Suite 310,
Sherman Oaks, CA 91403
(818) 905-0040

American Alliance of Health, Physical Education, Recreation, and Dance
1900 Association Dr., Reston, VA 22091
(703) 476-3400

American College of Sports Medicine
401 W. Michigan St.,
Indianapolis, IN 46206
(317) 637-9200

American Heart Association
7320 Greenville Ave., Dallas, TX 75231
(214) 750-5300

American Red Cross
18th & D Streets, N.W., Washington, DC 20006
(703) 379-8160

Aquatic Exercise Association
P. O. Box 497, Port Washington, WI 53074
(414) 375-2503 or (800) 545-4141

Association for Fitness in Business
965 Hope St., Stamford, CT 06907
(203) 359-2188

Athletic Institute
200 Castlewood Dr., No. Palm Beach, FL 33408
(305) 842-4100

Body Architects, Inc.
10 James Street, East Providence, RI 02914
(401) 431-2115

Excellence in Exercise Association
29 Vespa Lane, Nashua, NH 03060
(603) 882-6780

Exer-Safety Association
2044 Euclid Ave., Cleveland, OH 44115
(216) 687-1718

Institute For Aerobics Research
12200 Preston Rd., Dallas, TX 75230
(800) 635-7050

International Dance Exercise Association
6190 Cornerstone Court E., San Diego, CA 92121
(619) 535-8979

International Racquet Sports Association
132 Brookline Ave., Boston, MA 02215
(617) 236-1500

International School of Aerobic Training
5555 Cloud Way, San Diego, CA 92117
(619) 571-8890

Jazzercise®
2080 Roosevelt, Carlsbad, CA 92008
(619) 434-2101

National Dance Exercise Instructor's Training Association
1503 S. Washington Ave., Suite 208,
Minneapolis, MN 55454
(800) 237-6242

National Handicapped Sports and Recreation Association
Farragut Station, P. O. Box 33141,
Washington, DC 20033
(202) 783-1441

National Injury Prevention Foundation
8575 Gibbs Ave., #109, San Diego, Ca 92123
(619) 480-8200

National Institute For Fitness and Sport
250 N. Agnes St., Indianapolis, IN 46202
(317) 274-3432

National Strength and Conditioning Association
251 Capitol Beach Blvd., Lincoln, NE 68528
(402) 472-3000

Personal Fitness and Bodywork Professionals Association
121 W. 17th St., #8D, New York, NY 10011
(212) 620-4321

President's Council on Physical Fitness and Sports
450 Fifth St., N.W., Washington, DC 20001
(202) 272-3430

Jacki Sorensen's Aerobic Program/AKA Aerobic Dancing
18907 Nordhoff St., Northridge, CA 91328
(818) 885-0032

Equipment

Stationery and Outdoor Bikes/ Recumbent Bikes

Bodyguard
40 Radio Circle, Mt. Kisco, NY 10549
(800) 828-1186

Dynavit of America
23832 Rockfield Blvd., #265
Lake Forest, CA 92630
(714) 583-1707

Exercycle Corp.
667 Providence St., Woonsocket, RI 02895
(800) 367-6712

Heart-Mate
260 W. Beach Ave., Inglewood, CA 90302
(213) 674-5030

Kidcycle
13348 Grass Valley Ave., Grass Valley, CA 95945
(916) 477-2500

Life Fitness
9601 Jeronimo Rd., Irvine, CA 92718
(800) 643-8637

Maximus Fitness Products
208 E. 2nd Ave., La Habra, CA 90631
(213) 694-0800

Paramount
6450 E. Bandini Blvd., Los Angeles, CA 90040
(800) 521-2121

Performance USA
106 Regal Row, Dallas, TX 75247
(800) 292-5666

Precor
P. O. Box 3004, Bothell, WA 98041
(206) 486-9292

Pro-Tech
1965 E. Blair, Santa Ana, CA 92705
(800) 453-5332

Schwinn
615 Landwehr Rd., Northbrook, IL 60062
(312) 291-9100

Floors & Mats

Aerobafloor
9540 E. Jewel St., Parker Plaza, Denver, CO 80231
(303) 745-5305

Aerobisport
9319 E. Harry, Wichita, KS 67207
(316) 687-4489

American Athletic
200 American Ave.; Jefferson, IA 50129
(515) 386-3125

Athletic Spring Floor
221 Phlox St., Redlands, CA 92373

Connor Forest Industries
3361 Boyington Dr., Suite 180
Carrollton, TX 75006
(800) 972-1082

Diversified Products
P. O. Box 100, Opelika, AL 36803
(205) 749-9001

Duragrid, Inc.
840 W. 2500 South, Salt Lake City, UT 84119
(800) 421-8112

Exerflex
6786 Hawthorn Park Dr., Indianapolis, IN 46220
(317) 849-6181

Gerstung Fitness Floors
6310 Blair Hill Lane, Baltimore, MD 21209
(301) 337-7781

Kendall USA
2900 Horseshoe Dr. South, Naples, FL 33941
(813) 774-4808

Linray International
127 Airport Rd., Hyannis, MA 02601
(617) 778-1667

Mateflex
1712 Erie St., Utica, NY 13503
(800) 635-6353

Robbins, Inc.
P. O. Box 44238, Cincinnati, OH 45244
(513) 871-8988

Sentinel Fitness Products
130 North St., Hyannis, MA 02601
(617) 775-5220

Sports and Fitness Products
P. O. Box 1307, Cartersville, GA 30120
(404) 382-7718

Stage Step
P. O. Box 328, Philadelphia, PA 19105
(215) 567-6662

Tiger America
2215 York Rd., Ste. 108, Oakbrook, IL 60521
(312) 990-1222

Torin, Inc.
9 Industrial Park, Waldwick, NJ 07463
(800) 634-6650

USA Products
P. O. Box 546, Gardner, KS 66030
(913) 888-5755

Ultimate Aerobic Floor
2301 N. W. 33rd Ct., Pompano Beach, FL 33069
(305) 978-1700

Weights—Hand/Ankle

American Athletic Inc.
200 American Ave., Jefferson, IA 50129
(800) 247-3978

Diversified Products
P. O. Box 100, Opelika, AL 36801
(205) 749-9001

Elmer's
P. O. Box 16326, Lubbock, TX 79490
(800) 858-4568

Excel
9935 Beverly Blvd., Pico Rivera, CA 90660
(213) 699-0311

Fitness Dimensions
1280-B Lambert Rd., Brea, CA 92621
(213) 690-4152

Gymjazz
3119 W. Burbank Blvd., Burbank, CA 91505
(818) 954-0077

Han-Teens
P. O. Box 18510, Spokane, WA 99208
(509) 326-5470

Hardbody Fitness Systems
22600-B Lambert, #807, El Toro, CA 92630
(714) 768-8070

Lin-Ray International
127 Airport Rd., Hyannis, MA 02601
(617) 778-1667

NDL Products
2205 N.W. 30th Place, Pompano Beach, FL 33060
(800) 843-3021

Soft-Weights
3131 Western Ave., Seattle, WA 98121
(206) 282-3031

Spenco
P. O. Box 2501, Waco TX 76702
(817) 772-6000

Triangle Health & Fitness
P. O. Box 2000, Morrisville, NC 27560
(919) 469-4111

Vig Industries Inc.
2050 Clark Drive, Vancouver, B.B. VSN3G7
(800) 663-7743

Whitely Fitness
135 S. Washington Ave., Bergenfield, NJ 07621
(201) 384-9711

Bands/Tubing

Aerobics Power Bands
6065 Mission Gorge Rd., San Diego, CA 92120
(619) 462-2413

Hygienic Corp.
1245 Home Ave., Akron, OH 44310
(216) 633-8460

Spri Products
962 Northwest Hwy, Park Ridge, IL 60068
(800) 222-7774

Charts

Anatomical Chart Co.
7124 N. Clark St., Chicago, IL 60626
(312) 764-5445

Pro-Fit
P. O. Box 2339, Kirkland, WA 98083
(206) 367-6287

Pulse
2221 E. Somerset, Salt Lake City, UT 84121
(801) 943-6738

Workout Warehouse
7724 So. Silver Lake Drive
Salt Lake City, UT 84121
(801) 942-8437

Treadmills

Heart Rate
3186-G Airway Ave., Costa Mesa, CA 92626
(800) 237-2271

Pacer Industries
1121 Crowley Rd., Carrollton, TX 75006
(214) 446-3535

Precor
P. O. Box 3004, Bothell, WA 98041
(800) 662-0606

Stairmaster
259 Route 17, Newburgh, NY 12550
(800) 772-0089

Books

Physiology and Kinesiology

Exercise in Health and Disease
Pollock, Wilmore, and Fox. W. B. Saunders,
W. Washington Square, Philadelphia, PA 19105
(215) 574-4700

Exercise Physiology
McArdle, Katch and Katch. Lea & Febiger
600 Washington Square
Philadelphia, PA 19106-4198
(215) 922-1330

Guidelines for Exercise Testing and Prescription
American College of Sports Medicine. Lea &
Febiger, 600 Washington Square
Philadelphia, PA 19106-4198
(215) 922-1330

Kinesiology and Applied Anatomy
Rasch and Burke. Lea & Febiger,
600 Washington Square
Philadelphia, PA 19106-4198
(215) 922-1330

Kinesiology: Scientific Basis of Human Motion
Wells and Luttgens. W. B. Saunders, W. Washington Square, Philadelphia, PA 19105
(215) 574-4700

Physiology of Fitness
Sharkey Athletic Institute,
200 Castlewood Dr., N. Palm Beach, FL 33408
(305) 842-3030

Stretch & Strengthen
Alter. Houghton Mifflin Co.
2 Park St., Boston, MA 02108
(617) 725-5000

Special Populations

Aquatics for Special Populations
YMCA Human Kinetics Publishers
Box 5076, Champaign, IL 61820

Children and Exercise XII
Brinkhorst, et al. Human Kinetics
Publishers, Inc.
Box 5076
Champaign, IL 61820
(217) 351-5076

Diabetics Guide to Health and Fitness
Berg. Human Kinetics Publishers, Inc.
Box 5076, Champaign, IL 61820
(217) 351-5076

Exercise In Pregnancy
Artal and Wiswell. Williams and Wilkins,
428, Preston St., Baltimore, MD 21202
(301) 528-4000

Fitness After 50
LaLanne. Stephen Greene Press, Viking
Penguin, Inc.
40 W. 23rd St., New York, NY 10010
(212) 337-5200

Seniors on the Move
Rikkers. Human Kinetics Publishers, Inc.
Box 5076, Champaign, IL 61820
(217) 351-5076

Sports Medicine

The Complete Book of Sports Medicine
Dominguez Athletic Institute
200 Castlewood Dr., N. Palm Beach, FL 33408
(305) 842-3030

Sports Injuries—Prevention and Treatment
Peterson and Renstrom.
Year Book Medical Publishers
35 E. Wacker Dr., Chicago, IL 60601
(312) 726-9733

The Sports Medicine Book
Mirkin and Hoffman. Little, Brown & Company
34 Beacon St., Boston MA 02106
(617) 227-0730

The Sports Medicine Fitness Course
Nieman. Bull Publishing Co.
P. O. Box 208, Palo Alto, CA 94302
(415) 322-2855

Standard First Aid and Personal Safety
2nd E., American National Red Cross.
Doubleday and Co.
501 Franklin Ave., Garden City. NY 11530
(516) 294-4000

Your Injury: A Common Sense Guide to Sports Injuries
Ritter and Albohm. Benchmark Press
8435 Keystone Crossing, Indianapolis, IN 46240

Footwear

Adidas USA
15 Independence Blvd., Warren, NJ 07060
(201) 580-0700

ASICS Tiger
3030 S. Susan St., Santa Ana, CA 92704
(714) 754-0451

Autry
11420 Reeder Rd., Dallas, TX 75229
(214) 241-7793

Avia
16160 S.W. Upper Boones Ferry Rd.,
Portland, OR 97224
(800) 547-3213

Brooks
9341 Courtland Dr., Rockford, MI 49351
(616) 874-8448

Converse
One Fordham Rd., No. Reading, MA 01864
(617) 664-0194

Ellesse
1430 Broadway, 18th Floor, New York, NY 10018
(212) 840-6111

Etonic
147 Centre St., Brockton, MA 02403
(617) 583-9033

Foot-Joy
144 Field St., Brockton, MA 02403
(617) 586-2233

Kaepa
5410 Kaepa Ct., San Antonio, TX 78218
(512) 661-7463

Kangaroos
1809 Clarkson Rd., Chesterfield, MO 63017
(314) 532-3357

L.A. Gear
4221 Redwood Ave., Los Angeles, CA 90066
(213) 822-1995

Lotto USA
2301 McDaniel Dr., Carrollton, TX 75006
(214) 351-2537

New Balance
38 Everett St., Boston, MA 02134
(617) 783-4000

Nike
9000 S.W. Nimbus Dr., Beaverton, OR 97005
(503) 644-9000

Pony
201 Route 17 North, Rutherford, NJ 07070
(201) 896-0101

Puma
492 Old Connecticut Path
Framingham, MA 01701
(617) 875-0660

Reebok
150 Royall St., Canton, MA 02021
(617) 821-2800

Ryca
36 Finnell Dr., Weymouth, MA 02188
(617) 331-8800

Saucony
Centennial Industrial Park, Centennial Dr.
Peabody, MA 01961
(617) 532-9000

Tretorn
147 Centre St., Brockton, MA 02403
(617) 583-9100

Turntec
16542 Milliken Ave., Irvine, CA 92714
(714) 474-4974

Music and Videos

Music

Aerobic Beat
7985 Santa Monica Blvd., #109
Los Angeles, CA 90046
(213) 659-2503

Aerobic Connection
P. O. Box 4612, Carlsbad, CA 92008
(800) 832-2448

Aerobic Dance Music
324 S. Maple Ave., Oakpark, IL 60302
(312) 848-3959

Aerobics Records
2055 Edinburg, Cardiff, CA 92007
(619) 943-1649

Aerobitech
27417 Onlee Ave., Saugus, CA 91350
(800) 468-7428

ASCAP
1 Lincoln Plaza, New York, NY 10023
(212) 870-7576

BMI
320 W. 57th St., New York, NY 10019
(800) 872-2641

David Shelton Productions
780 E. 315 S. Layton, UT 84041
(801) 544-0583

Disco Beats
17 Old Route 146 Clifton, NY 12065
(518) 371-5555

East Coast Music Productions
P. O. Box 3812, Gaithersburg, MD 20878
(800) 777-BEAT

JDL Records, Inc.
567 W. 5th St., San Pedro, CA 90731
(213) 519-7393

Music Mixes
2934 Northwood Blvd., Orlando, FL 32803
(407) 644-5322

Postmark Records
614 Fell, San Francisco, CA 94102
(415) 431-5358

Seniors Records
18455 Burbank Blvd., Ste. 412, Tarzana, CA 91355

Supreme Audio
271 Greenway Rd., Ridgewood, NJ 07450
(201) 445-7398

TSR Records
8335 Sunset Blvd., Los Angeles, CA 90069
(213) 656-0970

12" Dance Records
2010 P St. N.W., Washington, DC 20036
(202) 659-2010

Videos

Aerobics on the Easy Side (Dr. Jean Rosenbaum)
Vista Vision, P. O. Box 1429, Durango, CO 81301
(800) 843-3611

American College of Obstetricians and Gynecologists
Feeling Fine Programs, Inc.
3575 Cahuenga Blvd. West, #440,
Los Angeles, CA 90068
(213) 850-6400

The Ballet Workout
Instructional Video
P. O. Box 757, Bloomington, IN 47402
(800) 255-8989

Best Fat Burners
AFAA, 15250 Ventura Blvd., Suite 310,
Sherman Oaks, CA 91403
(818) 905-0040

Bodies in Motion
P. O. Box 88046, Honolulu, HI 98630
(808) 527-4911

Body Focus (Richard Wilson)
Video Takes, Lackwanna Plaza
Montclair, NJ 07042

The Bodysculpture System (Beth Johnson, Tina Plakinger)
Video Takes, Lackwanna Plaza
Montclair, NJ 07042

Creative Instructors Aerobics
C.I.A., 2314 Naudain St., Philadelphia, PA 19146
(800) 435-0055

CPR For Everyone
Double A Productions, Evergreen Way
Stratham, NH 03885
(603) 778-3010

Esquire Great Body Series (Deborah Crocker)
2 Park Ave., New York, NY 10016
(212) 561-8100

David Essel's Beach Workout
2353 Periwinkle Way, Sanibel Island, FL 33957
(800) 222-7774

Exercise Essentials (Sue Thompson)
Sue Thompson Inc., 116 W. Eastman, #204
Arlington Heights, IL 60004-5938
(312) 255-2425

Exercise Shorts (Madeleine Lewis, Chet Vienne)
Karl-Lorimar Home Video
17942 Cowan Ave., Irvine, CA 92714
(714) 474-0355

The Complete Guide to Exercise Videos (Catalog)
Collage Video
5398 Main St., N.E., Minneapolis, MN 55421
(800) 433-6769

The Firm: Workout with Weights
Meridian Films
P. O. Box 5917, Columbia, SC 29250
(803) 799-6239

Fit To Be Tried (Melanie Kirk-Stauffer)
P. O. Box 8355, Tacoma, WA 98408
(800) 445-4494, Ext. 1045

Fitness Is For Everyone
National Handicapped Sports and
Recreation Association
24 Public Square, Cleveland, OH 44113

Fitness Over 50
Health Tapes, Inc.
13225 Capital Ave., Oak Park, MI 48237
(313) 548-2500

Freedanse I and II
M.T.I. Homevideo
14352 S.W. 142 Ave., Miami, FL 33186
(800) 821-7461

Gymboree
Lorimar Home Video
17942 Cowan, Irvine, CA 92714
(714) 474-0355

Jammin' With Johnny
Awasvideo, P. O. Box 3319,
No. Las Vegas, NV 89030

Jump To It
Jump To It Productions
11902 Los Coyotes, La Mirada, CA 90638
(213) 943-4017

Just Steps
Smooth Moves
225 N. Congress, #332, Austin, TX 78701
(512) 237-5222

The Low Impact/No Stress Workout
AFAA
15250 Ventura Blvd., Suite 310
Sherman Oaks, CA 91403
(818) 905-0040

L.A. Workout (Candace Copeland)
1849 Sawtelle Blvd., #101
Los Angeles, CA 90025

National Aerobics Championship Workout
General Foods Corp.
P. O. Box 4886, Kankakee, IL 60902
(312) 278-9700

One On One (Linda Shelton)
Fit Video
9540 E. Jewell, Suite A, Denver, CO 80231
(800) 445-5262

Panaerobics
Powerhouse, 23 W. Anapahu
Santa Barbara, CA 93101
(805) 966-7527

Pregnancy: The Aerobic Way
Bonnie Rote
2206 S. Cherry, Mesa, AZ 85202

Principles and Techniques of Dance-Exercise Choreography
Brick Bodies, 212 W. Padonia Rd.
Timonium, MD 21093
(301) 252-5280

Shape Up I & II (Sandy & Kyle Zook)
Ortho-Sport
P. O. Box 22178, Phoenix, AZ 85028
(602) 971-1109

Stay Fit Rebounding
Fit For You, 2377 S. Hacienda Blvd.
Hacienda Heights, CA 91745
(818) 369-2021

Toning The Total Body
AFAA, 15250 Ventura Blvd., Suite 310
Sherman Oaks, CA 91403
(818) 905-0040

Tamilee Webb's Rubber Band Workout
Feeling Fine Products
3575 Cahuenga Blvd. West, Suite 440
Los Angeles, CA 90068
(213) 332-3373

Sit and Reach Box

Construction

1. Using any sturdy wood or comparable construction material (3/4 inch plywood or comparable construction material is recommended), cut the following pieces:
   2 pieces—12 in. x 12 in.
   2 pieces—12 in. x 10 in.
   1 piece—12 in. x 21 in.
2. Assemble the pieces using nails or screws, and wood glue.

3. Inscribe the top panel with one centimeter gradations. It is crucial that the 23 centimeter line be exactly in line with the vertical plane against which the subject's feet will be placed.
4. Cover the apparatus with two coats of polyurethane sealer or shellac.
5. For convenience, a handle can be made by cutting a 1 in. x 3 in. hole in the top panel.
6. The measuring scale should extend from about 9 to 50 cm.

Constructing the sit and reach box

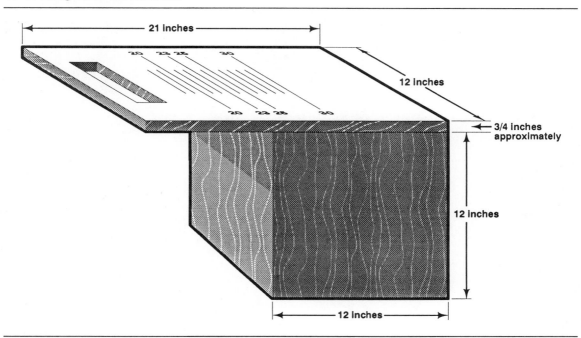

APPENDIX H

Miscellaneous

Insurance Companies

Rhulen Agency (Liability)
217 Broadway, Monticello, NY 12701
(914) 794-8000

Baldinger Insurance (Health)
100 Wilshire Blvd., #450
Santa Monica, CA 90401
(213) 394-BFIT

GLOSSARY

Aerobic Terms

Abduction is moving a body segment, such as arm or leg, away from the center of the body (such as raising one's arms from a position along side the body to an angle straight out from the shoulder).

Adduction is bringing the body segment back to the center of the body (such as bringing arms back towards the body).

Aerobic refers to the use of oxygen by the body for a sustained activity of two minutes or longer.

Aerobic capacity (cardiorespiratory endurance) is the ability of the body to remove oxygen from the air and transfer it through the lungs and blood to the working muscles.

Aerobic dance exercise is a form of exercise that incorporates a variety of dance movements performed to motivating music.

Aerobics is a popular form of exercise that incorporates vigorous, bouncy movements and locomotor movements to provide a fun form of fitness development and exercise.

Agonist is the muscle contracting concentrically (such as the biceps in a curl).

Alignment refers to the correct positioning of the spine and the body parts. Alignment has postural implications (refers to how all the body parts line up).

Amino acids, the building blocks of protein, are organic compounds containing nitrogen, hydrogen, and carbon.

Anaerobic means without oxygen; usually refers to the body's ability to perform short-spurt, high-energy activities, such as sprinting, without the need for oxygen replenishment.

Arteriosclerosis is the abnormal thickening or hardening of the arteries which causes the inner artery walls to lose their elasticity.

Artery is the large vessel that carries oxygenated blood away from the heart to the body tissues.

Atherosclerosis is a general term for a disease that leads to the thickening and hardening of the inner layer of the artery wall due to fat deposits. It causes a decrease in the inner diameter of the artery.

Ballistic movements are jerky, bouncy, explosive, and unsustained movements.

Basal Metabolic Rate is the sum total of energy required by all the physiologic processes required to maintain life; the number of calories burned to sustain life.

Blood pooling refers to a condition caused by ceasing vigorous exercise too abruptly so that blood remains in the extremities and may not be delivered quickly enough to the heart and brain.

Blood pressure refers to the amount of pressure the blood exerts against the walls of the arteries during each heart contraction and heart relaxation. Taking the blood pressure measures the pressure of the blood in the arteries.

Body alignment is how the torso, limbs, spine, shoulders, head, etc. are positioned. Proper body alignment refers to the optimal placement and posture of the body during exercise to ensure safe, injury-free movement.

Body composition is the proportion of body fat to lean body mass (muscle, bone, cartilage, vital organs). Proper body composition is a part of overall fitness.

Calorie is the common word used to refer to the kilocalorie. A kilocalorie is a measure of the value of foods that produce heat and energy in the body. One calorie is equal to the amount of heat required to raise the temperature of one gram of water one degree Centigrade.

Carbohydrate refers to organic compounds containing carbon, hydrogen, and oxygen. When broken down, carbohydrates are the main energy source for muscular work and one of the basic foodstuffs in the diet.

Carotid pulse is the pulse located on the carotid artery just under the jawbone. It is the common area used for taking the heart rate during and following exercise, as it is quick and easy to locate.

Cardiovascular efficiency refers to the ability of the body to deliver oxygen to all of its vital organs efficiently during the stress of exercise.

Cholesterol is a chemical compound found in animal fats and oils. High levels of cholesterol in the blood are often associated with a high risk of atherosclerosis.

Chronic refers to something persisting over a long period of time.

Coronary arteries are the two main arteries arising from the aorta and arching down over the top of the heart. They are the major arteries responsible for carrying blood to the heart muscle.

Diastolic pressure is blood pressure within the arteries when the heart is in relaxation between contractions.

Duration is the length of time devoted to an exercise or an exercise session.

Ectomorph is a body type or somatotype. This type of person appears thin and lean.

Empty calories refers to food which yields calories that are void or nearly void of nutrients, protein, vitamins, and minerals. This usually refers to foods having high sugar or fat content, and alcoholic beverages.

Endomorph is a body type or somatotype. This type of person appears soft and round with a predominance of fat tissue, but is not necessarily obese.

Extension is increasing the angle of a joint (such as straightening your arms from a bent position).

Fat is stored in the body as adipose tissue. It serves as a concentrated source of energy for muscular work; a compound containing glycerol and fatty acids.

Fatigue refers to a diminished capacity for work as a result of prolonged or excessive exertion.

Flexibility is the ability of the joint to move through its full range of motion.

High-impact is a form of aerobics that incorporates jumping and bouncing movements. There is a high degree of impact placed on the joints, bones, and feet in this form of aerobic classes.

Hyperextension is when the angle of a joint is moved past the normal range of motion.

Intensity is the level of difficulty of an exercise or workout.

Lordosis refers to an increased lumbar curve or "sway back."

Low-impact is a form of aerobics that keeps one foot on the floor at all times; often refers to aerobic classes that involve no jumping.

Low Intensity means a reduced workload, or working at a lower target heart rate.

Metabolism is the chemical reaction of a cell or living tissue that transfers usable materials into energy.

Mesomorph is a somatotype or body type describing the very muscular, athletic-looking individual.

Muscular endurance is the ability of the muscles to exert force over an extended period of time.

Muscular strength is the amount of force produced when a muscle group contracts and moves a resistance.

Overload is the method used to increase the workload beyond the normal capacity to improve and develop muscular strength and endurance.

Overuse syndrome refers to slow-to-heal, nagging ailments that result from exercising too much, too soon; can involve muscles, tendons, or bones; respond to a treatment of rest, ice, compression, and elevation (RICE).

Nautilus is a type of weight machine that uses special cams to change the amount of force needed to lift the weight so that the muscle is working closer to maximum throughout the exercise.

Perceived exertion is a means of measuring how hard one is exercising by comparing a subjective self-rating with an established chart of various levels.

Prone is lying face down.

Radial artery is the artery located on the inside of the wrist. It lies very close to the surface of the skin and is therefore often used for counting the pulse.

Recovery Heart Rate is how quickly your pulse returns to normal after an aerobic workout.

Repetition is one complete action of an exercise.

Resting Heart Rate refers to the number of times your heart beats per minute when you have been sitting or resting for approximately 10 minutes.

RICE is the acronym for rest, ice, compress, elevate: the steps for immediate injury treatment.

Risk factors refers to genetics and nongenetic characteristics that contribute to the incidence of heart disease or stroke.

Static stretching movements place the muscle in a sustained stretch position for a given period of time. This is an effective way to achieve flexibility in a specific muscle group. It is the opposite of ballistic stretching movements.

Set-Point Theory proposes that human metabolism works very hard to maintain a certain body weight; that weight is held in place through complex homeostatic mechanisms.

Shin splints is a catch-all phrase used to describe any discomfort in the front lower leg. Usually a result of overuse syndrome.

Side stitch refers to a pain in the side during exercise. It is thought to be caused by a spasm in the diaphragm, due to insufficient oxygen supply and improper breathing.

Sprain refers to a wrenching or twisting of a joint in which ligaments are stretched past their normal limits.

Strain refers to a "muscle pull," a stretch or a tear of the muscle or adjacent tissue.

Strength is the maximum force or tension that a muscle or muscle group can produce against a resistance.

Supine is lying face up.

Target Heart Rate is the level at which you will gain the benefits of exercising your heart to improve cardiovascular fitness.

Tendon is a band of dense, fibrous tissue forming the termination of a muscle and attaching muscle to bone with a minimum of elasticity.

Tendinitis is inflammation of a tendon; often requires several weeks of rest to completely heal.

Time refers to the length of time devoted to a workout, a class, or a particular exercise.

Training effects are the physiologic adaptations that occur as a result of aerobic exercise of sufficient intensity, frequency, and duration to produce beneficial changes in the body.

Triglycerides are compounds composed of glycerol fatty acids. They are stored in the body and are unhealthy when in high levels.

Vein is a vessel carrying blood away from the body and toward the heart.

Vertebrae are the bony or cartilaginous segments that are separated by discs and make up the spinal column.

Warm-up is a balanced combination of static stretch and rhythmic limbering exercises that prepare the body for more vigorous exercise.

Working heart rate is the heart rate taken at the end of the aerobic section of a workout to identify whether the individual was working in his or her target heart rate zone and at the proper intensity for age and physical fitness level.

INDEX

Abdominal curl-ups, 38–39
Abductor, 40, 68
Achilles' tendinitis, 24, 64
Adductor, 41, 68
Aerobic capacity, *See* Cardiovascular
    endurance
Aerobic dance exercise, 2, 3, 20–21, 28, 62
Aerobic exercise,
    benefits, 6, 20
    components, 20–23
    definition, 2, 28
    formula, 2
    goals, 49
    low-impact, 76, 79–80, 86, 106
    mental benefits, 48–49
    results, 3
    shoes, 24–26, 77
    water, 79
Alignment, body, 66–67
    and pregnancy, 83
American College of Sports Medicine, 10
Amino acids, 55
Angina, 16
Ankle circles, 34, 35
Ankle raises, 34, 35
Artery, carotid, 8
Asthma, 73
Atherosclerosis, 16
Ballistic movements, 22
Basal metabolic rate, 57, 79
Blood pooling, 23
Blood pressure, 13–16
Body composition, 7, 57
Body types, 7
Buttocks exercise, 42
Calorie, 6, 20, 49, 54–58
    empty, 54
Can-Can kick, 113
Carbohydrates, 54
Cardiac risk, 73
Cardiovascular
    disease, 12–16, 73

efficiency, 6, 8, 24
    endurance, 6, 8
Cardiovascular work
    during pregnancy, 84
Carotid pulse, 8
Certification, 120–121
Charleston Bounce Step, 113
Chest pain, 73
Cholesterol, 6, 57
Chronic, 64
Clothing, 24
Cool down, 22–23
    during pregnancy, 85
Coronary arteries, 6, 16
Coronary atherosclerosis, 16
CPR, 98
Diastolic pressure, *See* Blood pressure
Dizziness, 22, 23, 73
    during pregnancy, 87
Duration, 12
Ectomorph, 7
Electrical impedance, 57
Endomorph, 7
Endorphins, 20, 48
Enkephalin, 20
EVA (ethylene vinyl acetate), 24
Exercise
    duration of, 12
    frequency, 11–12
    intensity of, 12
    intolerance, 73
    overload, 8
Exercises
    strengthening, 37–42
    isolations, 28–37
    stretches, 28–37
    to avoid, 70–72
    warm-up, 28–37
Fat, 3, 6, 7, 15, 16, 54, 55, 56–57
Fatigue, 10, 66, 78, 90
Fever, 73
Fiber, 54–55

Fitness, 2, 8
  components of, 6
Flexibility, 7, 22–23, 90, 94
Floors, 65, 66, 67, 77, 99
Floorwork, 22
  during pregnancy, 84–85
Footwear, *See* Shoes
Glycogen, 54
Grapevine, 114
Grapevine Schottische, 115
Heat, 72
Heart, 8
Heart rate
  monitoring, 11
Heel walking, 34, 35
High-impact, 106
  and pregnancy, 87
Hip circles, 31
Hives, 73
Humidity, 72
Hydration, 56
Hydrastatic weighing, 57
Hyperextension, 37, 70, 77, 78
Injuries
  causes, 64–73
  knee, 64
  overuse, 63–64, 76–77
  prevention of, 62–63
Intensity, 10, 11, 12, 21, 22, 24, 47, 72, 79, 80, 99
Isolations, 28–31
  head, 28, 29
  hip, 30, 31
  rib, 28, 30
Jaw pain, 73
Karvonen Method, 10
Kegels, 86
Knee injuries, 64
Knee lifts
  during pregnancy, 87
Knee protection, 77
Leg lifts, 39–41
LIA *See* Low-impact aerobics
Light-headedness, 73
Lower back precautions, 77
Low-impact aerobics, 86, 106
  benefits, 79–80
  definition, 76, 79
Low-intensity, 79
Lunges, 32

Mesomorph, 7
Metabolism, 6, 20, 56, 56, 79
Minerals, 56
Modified Step Test, 92–93
Motivation, 46
  inner-directed, 47–48
  negative,46–47
  outer-directed, 48
  positive, 47
Mountain Climber, 111
Muscles, 67–69
Muscular endurance, 7
Muscular strength, 7
Music, 104
Nausea, 73
Negative motivation, 46–47
Nutrition, 54–56
Overload, 7, 8
Overuse syndrome, 46, 62–65
Pain
  arm, 73
  jaw, 73
Palpitations, 73
Pelvic lifts, 42
Perceived exertion, 84
Plantar fasciitis, 63
Pony, 111
Positive motivation, 47
Prone, 88
Protein, 55
Pulse, 8, 9
  at the carotid artery, 8
  at the radial artery, 9
  irregular, 73
Push-ups, 37–38
Radial artery, 9
Recovery heart rate, 8, 11
Repetition, 7, 43, 78, 86
Resistance, 7
Resting heart rate, 8
Rib circles, 30
RICE, 62–63, 64
Ringing in ears, 73
Risk factors, 6, 8, 12–16, 73
RISKO, 13–16
Schottische, 114
Set-point theory, 56
Shin splints, 12, 64
Shoes, 24–26, 77
  improper, 65

Shortness of breath, 73
Shoulder circles, 28, 29
Sit and Reach Test, 94
Skiers' jump, 117
Somatotypes, 7
Sorenson, Jacki, 2
Standing work
   during pregnancy, 86–87
Static stretching, 21–22, 23
Strengthening exercises, 37–42
Stress, 6
Stress fractures, 64
Stress reactions, 64
Stretches, 32–37
  calf, 34
  hamstring, 33
  quadricep, 33
Stretching, 21–22
  ballistic, 70
  non-ballistic, 70
Target Heart Rate (THR), 8–10
  during pregnancy, 84
Torque, 77, 87
Training errors, 64–65

Triglyceride, 57
Video catalogs, 104
Videotapes, 102–104
Visualization, 49–50
Vitamins, 56
Vomiting, 73
Warm-up, 21–22
  pre-class, 28–37
  during pregnancy, 82–83
Water, 56
Weight control, 6, 56–57
Weight loss, 58
Weight table
  for men, 13
  for women, 14
Weights, 65, 78–79, 99
  during pregnancy, 87
Workout
  cardiovascular, 22
  clothing, 24
  frequency, 24
  results, 24
  strengthening and toning, 22